Walked out of the new road to conquer cancer 6 （六）(Vol. 6)
(The new concept of XZ-C cancer prevention and treatment)

BUILD UP THE MULTIDISCIPLINARY AND THE SCIENCE CITY OF THE RESEARCH BASE

with

RELATED TO CANCER RESEARCH FOR CONQUERING CANCER

Promoting the New Progresses in Oncology in the 21st Century
How to conquer cancer?
How to treat cancer? How to prevent cancer?
Volume VI

Authors: Xu Ze (China); Xu Jie (China) ; Bin Wu (America)
Translators: Bin Wu ; Lily Xu ; Zihao Xu ; Bo Wu
Editors: Bin Wu, Lily Xu, Tao Wu
Illustrators : Lily Xu, Bin Wu

authorHOUSE®

AuthorHouse™
1663 Liberty Drive
Bloomington, IN 47403
www.authorhouse.com
Phone: 1 (800) 839-8640

Published by AuthorHouse   03/29/2019

ISBN: 978-1-7283-0622-3 (sc)
ISBN: 978-1-7283-0621-6 (e)

Library of Congress Control Number: 2019903694

Print information available on the last page.

Build up the multidisciplinary and the science city of research base with related to cancer research for conquering cancer

Promoting the new progresses in oncology in the 21st century

1. *Established the overall framework for conquering cancer, which is the only way to conquer cancer*
2. *Proposed the overall design, plan, program, blueprint and implementation rules of the Science City*
3. *Equivalent to designing the overall framework for Chinese characteristics to conquer cancer*
4. *The following is the implementation of XZ-C's outline of how to conquer cancer:*

The main project to implement the outline of how to conquer cancer is:

The Structural Work:

1. *Conquering cancer and launching the general attack of cancer, focusing on prevention and control and treatment at the same level and at the same attention and at the same time*
2. *Creating the multidisciplinary and cancer-related scientific research base – the Science City*

Two-wing projects:

A wing - *how to conquer cancer ? How to **prevent** cancer? - to **reduce the incidence** of cancer*

B wing - *how to overcome cancer? How to **treat** cancer? - to **improve cancer cure rate***

The Aims:

A: *Reduce the incidence of cancer*
B: *Improve cancer cure rate, **prolong patient survival, and improve patient quality of life***

If this overall design and planning blueprint of conquering cancer can be implemented and achieved, it is possible to overcome cancer.

How to implement, how to achieve this general guideline r, programs, plans, blueprints of conquering cancer?

It should be set up " the research group of conquering cancer and of launching the general attack of cancer."

Invite the famous experts, professors, academic leaders or leading scientists; the scientists, entrepreneurs,leaders and volunteers of supporting conquering cancer and launching the general attack ; invite them to work together to make an unprecedented event in human history, that is, "to conquer cancer and to launch the general attack of cancer," and "to create a science city that conquers cancer" for the benefit of mankind.

Prepare for construction:

"The first science city of the Scientific Research Base for conquering cancer in the nation"

"The first science city of the Scientific Research Base for conquering cancer in the world"

TABLE OF CONTENTS

Volume I

Volume II

INTRODUCTION TO THIS BOOK

Bin Wu and Lily Xu

Each time when the book is finished, tears are full of both of my eyes. Each word in these series of books represents hard work and time and dedication and care for human health. These series are not just written down but are worked down.

Science Life is not always smooth and sometimes is extremely difficult. Science is endless. ***Only those who are not afraid of failure or risk can reach the summit of the mountain.***

In medical history the Greek physician Hippocrates (460-370 BC), who is considered the "Father of Medicine", was credited to the origin of the name **Cancer**. He used the terms *carcinos* and *carcinoma* to recount non-ulcer forming and ulcer-forming tumors. In Greek, these words refer to a crab because the finger-like spreading projections from cancer were similar to the shape of a crab. In his books, there are some records which also were written down: *"Everyone has a physician inside him or her; we just have to help it in its work. The natural healing force within each of us is the **greatest** force in getting well. Let our food as our medicine, and let medicine be our food"*.

*What is **the physician** inside him or her? where is this physician in the body? Why is it the **greatest force** in getting well?*

Dr. Xu Zu *in China works very hard with the **superb surgical** skills and did many basis and clinical experiments to search for cancer pathogenesis and etiology and prevention of cancer and treatment of cancer and the relationship between immune function and cancer, especially he found that when the center immune organ Thymus is removed, the tumor-bearing animal model can be made or when the immune function is decreased by immunesupressant, the tumor-bearing animal model can be* made. Meanwhile, a series of medication productions were produced which have great basic and clinical effect after the decade verification by **Dr. Xu Ze**. In this book, there are the detail plans for cancer prevention and treatment, more than 90% of cancer can be prevented, all of these theories have our basic and clinical experimental data to support.

<u>**Dr. Xu Ze**</u> the first time proposed many of the new concepts and theories on cancer internationally which are all of his innovation scientific theories from his basic experiments and clinical practices. All of the new theories and plans and designs are the great gift and the contribution to all of the human being. *The innovation of the theories is the same importance as the innovation of technology* such as a German-born theoretical physicist **Albert Einstein** developed the theory *of relativity* which is one of the two pillars of modern physics and is known for its influence on the philosophy of science; an English mathematician and physicist and astronomer and theologian and author **Sir Isaac Newton** is widely recognized as one of the most influential scientists of all time and a key figure in the scientific revolution. His book Mathematical Principles of Natural Philosophy was the first published in 1687 and laid the foundations of classical mechanics and formulated *the laws of motion and universal gravitation* that formed the dominant scientific viewpoint until it was superseded by the theory of relativity in his book; an English naturalist and geologist and biologist **Charles Robert Darwin** is the best known for his contributions *to the science of evolution* and his proposition that all species of life have descended over time from common ancestors is widely accepted and considered a foundational concept in science. In brief, <u>**Dr. Xu Zu has proposed many innovative cancer therapies concepts**</u>, especially cancer metastasis mechanisms and immune regulation and control cancer treatment which are the great contribution to our human being *in his different monographs and in these series of monographs*. Also, as we are known, the innovation always faces the great challenge to the traditional concepts or things. It needs to take great courage to challenge the tradition. All of Dr. Xu Ze's new cancer treatment therapies in his monographs have the basic and clinical experimental and data supporting and come from his scientific research results. Once again, it is the great contribution to the human being and it can save the patient life.

This innovation can lead to the development and improvement and also can face this great challenge.

Technology is rapidly developing and many medical mysteries had the answer. One day I took my time to brush up on or to go over Nobel Prize in medicine in the past years. The Nobel Prize in Physiology or Medicine 2016 was awarded for the discoveries of mechanisms for autophagy which is the body's internal recycling process--- recycle our trash to build the new cells. The process is crucial for preventing cancerous growths, warding off infection, etc. The word autophagy originates from two Greek words meaning "self-eating" which refers to the process in which cellular junk is captured and sealed in sack-like membranes called autophagosomes. The sealed contents are transported to another structure called the lysosome to process for rebuild the new cell for the body. The Nobel Prize in Physiology or Medicine 2018 was awarded for the discovery of the inhibition negative immune regulation for cancer therapy. Immune regulation and control is closely related to cancer therapy. In Dr. Xu Ze's series of monographs, there are the detailed records of his basic and clinical experiments and his innovative concepts of cancer therapies, many of which is involving in immune regulation and control cancer therapies.

Due to finishing the book in such a short period of time with much new information, if there are any errors, please forgive us and please contact us if you have any feedback.

Lastly, let work together to keep cancer away from humanity.

Bin Wu and Lily Xu

03-08-2019 in Timonium, MD, USA

A BRIEF INTRODUCTION
TO THE FIRST AUTHOR

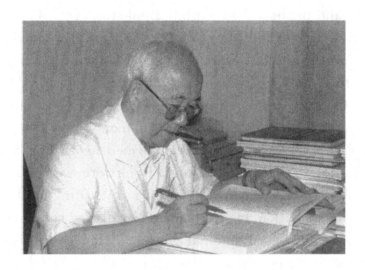

Xu Ze was born in 1933 in Leping City, Jiangxi Province, China. He graduated from Tongji Medical College in 1956. He served as the director of surgery, professor, chief physician, master and doctoral tutor of the Affiliated Hospital of Hubei College of Traditional Chinese Medicine. He is the director of the Experimental Surgery Research Institute of Hubei College of Traditional Chinese Medicine, director of the Department of Abdominal Oncology Surgery, and anti-cancer metastasis. Director of Recurrence Research Office; concurrently serves as executive director of Wuhan Branch of Chinese Medical Association, honorary president of Wuhan Anticancer Research Association, academic member of International Liver Disease Research Collaboration Center, member of International Federation of Surgeons, Chinese Journal of Experimental Surgery No. 1, 2, 3 The 4th Standing Editorial Board and the 1st, 2nd and 3rd Executive Editors of the Journal of Abdominal Surgery. He has been engaged in surgical work for 60 years and has extensive clinical experience in the surgical treatment of lung cancer, esophageal cancer, gastric cancer, liver cancer, gallbladder cancer, pancreatic cancer, and intestinal cancer, as well as the combination of Chinese and Western medicine to prevent postoperative recurrence and metastasis. In 1987, he began experimental research on tumors. Through cancer cell transplantation, he established tumor animal models, explored the mechanisms and rules of cancer metastasis and recurrence, and searched for ways to inhibit metastasis. Screening 48 kinds of natural drugs from anti-cancer invasion and metastasis And relapsed Chinese medicine, and based on this, developed xz-c immunomodulation anticancer traditional Chinese medicine preparation, clinically verified by a large number of cases, the effect is remarkable. Published 126 scientific research papers, published in 2001, "New Understanding and New Model of Cancer Treatment", published by Hubei Science and Technology Publishing House and published by Xinhua Bookstore. In 2006, he published the monograph "New Concept and New Method of Cancer Metastasis Treatment" published by Beijing People's Military Medical Publishing House and published by Xinhua Bookstore. In April 2007, he was awarded the original book award and certificate by the General Administration of Press and Publication of the People's Republic of China. In October 2011, the third monograph (New Concepts and New Methods of Cancer Treatment) was published by Beijing People's Military Medical Press. Xu Ze, Xu Jie/Zhang, Xinhua Bookstore was released. This book is translated into English by Dr. Bin Wu., published in Washington, DC on March 26, 2013, international distribution. He participated in 10 medical monographs such as "Hepatology Treatment" and "Abdominal Surgery". He engaged in teaching for 60 years, trained many young physicians, 10 master students And 2 doctoral students. He has been engaged in surgical research for 34 years and has achieved many results. Among them, "self-made xz-c: type abdominal cavity-venous bypass device for the treatment of cirrhotic refractory ascites and its clinical application" was awarded the Hubei Provincial Government Science and Technology for the second prize of the results, and promoted and applied in 38 hospitals across the country: The National Natural Science Foundation of China's experimental study on the pathophysiology and pathogenesis of pulmonary schistosomiasis by experimental surgical methods won the second prize of Hubei Provincial Government Science and Technology Achievements. He enjoys Special government allowance.

A BRIEF INTRODUCTION TO THE SECOND AUTHOR

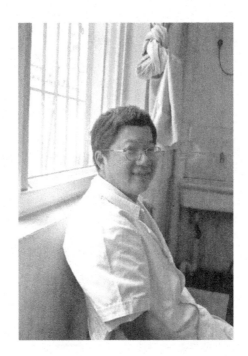

Xu Jie, male, graduated from Hubei College of Traditional Chinese Medicine in 1992, graduated from Hubei Medical University in 1996, Department of Clinical Medicine. Now He is chief physician in Hubei University of Traditional Chinese Medicine Hospital and Hubei Provincial Hospital of Surgery, engaged in experimental surgical tumor research and general surgery, urology clinical work.

Since 1992, he has been involved in the experimental tumor research of the Institute of Experimental Surgery of Hubei College of Traditional Chinese Medicine. He has carried out cancer cell transplantation and established a tumor animal model. He has carried out a series of experimental tumor research: exploring the mechanism of recurrence and metastasis of cancer and in vivo screening experiment of more than 200 kinds of Chinese herbal medicine in vivo tumor model of tumor inhibition s from a large number of natural medicine to find out, screening out of 48 kinds of anti-cancer invasion, metastasis, relapse traditional Chinese medicine

He participates in clinical validation and followed up for XZ - C immunoregulatory Chinese herbal medicine and completes the experimental research and clinical verification, data collection, collection and summary of this book.

A BRIEF INTRODUCTION TO THE THIRD AUTHOR AND THE MAIN TRANSLATOR AND THE MAIN EDITOR

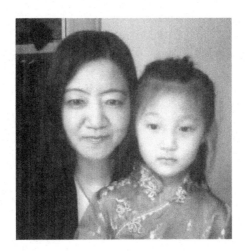

Bin Wu, MD, Ph.D., graduated from College of Yunyang of Tongji University of Medical Sciences for her MD degree; Studied her Master degree and her Ph. D degree in Sun Yat-Sen University of Medical Sciences. After she received her Ph.D., she worked as a Post-doctoral Follews in the Johns Hopkins Medical School and University of Maryland Medical School. She passed her USMLE tests and is going to do her residency training in America. She dedicated herself to oncology clinical and research. Her goal is to conquer cancer, which she believes this great contribution to our health. She has a daughter, named Lily Xu who drew all of the pictures in this book and is the great helper and gave the great ideas for Dr. Bin Wu.

A BRIEF INTRODUCTION TO THE ILLUSTRATOR AND THE ADVISOR

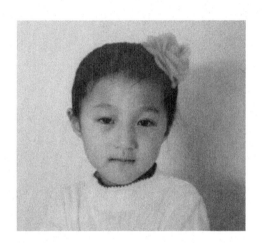

Lily Xu was born on November 17th 2006 and had an art presented in the Walter Art Museum in Baltimore at the age of 6; she got the fourth place trophy in the ES Double Digits or 24 and 24 games in the Baltimore County in Maryland; she got the first trophy in the BCPS STEM FAIR PHYSICS in Baltimore County; when she was in the sixth grade, she passed the advanced Math for 7th grade (which means the 8th grade math) test and moved the 8th grade math class; she loves the reading and writing and she finished many series of books. She got $6000 scholarship award for the Peabody music program in the Johns Hopkins University. In 2018 and 2019 she was chosen into Baltimore county Middle school Honor Band. In 2018 the robotic team which she attended for years got designing-award from the Baltimore county so that this robotic team came to Maryland State for the Robotic contest in 2019. On January 19th, 2019 she got the Robotic designing award in Maryland . She edits all of my books for the publishing and drew all of the pictures in this book. In 2019 she was chosen by Baltimore County for one duel and one ensemble to play Clarion.

THE MAIN TOPIC TO THIS BOOK

Under the guidance of Xi Jinping's new era of socialism with Chinese characteristics, we should strive to open up a new phase of scientific research in the new era, and the scientific research work to overcome cancer should be advanced.

Under the guidance of Xi Jinping's new era of socialism with Chinese characteristics, he strives to follow the path of self-innovation with Chinese characteristics and adheres to the road of independent innovation of "Chinese-style anti-cancer" combined with Chinese and Western medicine.

China will contribute more to the world's wisdom, China's programs, and China's power to overcome cancer. Let the sun of the human destiny community shine through the world.

Build up the Multidisciplinary and the Science City of Research Base with related to Cancer Research for Conquering Cancer

Promoting the new progress in oncology in the 21ˢᵗ century

How to conquer cancer?

How to treat cancer? How to prevent cancer?

Build up the Multidisciplinary and the Science City of Research Base with related to Cancer Research for Conquering Cancer

Promoting the new progresses in oncology in the 21st century

1. Established the overall framework for conquering cancer, which is the only way to conquer cancer
2. Proposed the overall design, plan, program, blueprint and implementation rules of Science City
3. Equivalent to designing the overall framework for Chinese characteristics to conquer cancer
4. The following is the implementation of XZ-C's outline of how to conquer cancer

The main project to implement the outline of how to overcome cancer is:

The Structural Work:

1. <u>Conquering cancer and launching the general attack of cancer, focusing on prevention, control, and treatment at the same level and at the same attention and at the same time</u>

2. <u>Creating the multidisciplinary and cancer-related scientific research base – the Science City</u>

Two-wing projects:

A wing - how to conquer cancer ? How to prevent cancer? - to reduce the incidence of cancer

B wing - how to overcome cancer? How to treat cancer? - to improve cancer cure rate

The Aims:

A: Reduce the incidence of cancer

B: Improve cancer cure rate, prolong patient survival, and improve patient quality of life

If this overall design and planning blueprint can be implemented and achieved of conquering cancer, it is possible to overcome cancer.

How to implement and how to achieve this general guideline, programs, plans, blueprints of conquering cancer?

It should be set up "the research group of conquering cancer and of launching the general attack ."

Invite the famous experts, professors, academic leaders or leading scientists; the scientists, entrepreneurs, leaders, and volunteers of supporting conquering cancer and launching the general attack ; invite them to work together to make an unprecedented event in human history, that is, "to overcome cancer and to launch the general attack of cancer," and "to create a science city that conquers cancer" for the benefit of mankind.

Prepare for construction:

"The first science city of the Scientific Research Base for conquering cancer in the nation"

"The first science city of the Scientific Research Base for conquering cancer in the world"

The library of Prevention of Cancer and Anti-cancer medical research

1. The Collected Works of Professor Xu Ze's Research on Cancer Prevention and Cancer Treatment

XZ-C proposed: How to overcome cancer? How to prevent cancer? How to treat cancer?

__XZ-C new concept of cancer treatment__

__*Volume I*__ *<<Conquer Cancer and Launch the total attack to cancer ——prevention cancer and cancer control and cancer treatment at the same level and at the same attention and at the same time>> The book table or contents or directory (omitted)*

__*Volume II*__ *<<Walked out of a new way of cancer treatment with the immune regulation and control of the combination of Chinese and Western medicine>> The book table or contents or directory (omitted)*

__*Volume III*__ *<<The research of XZ-C immunomodulation anticancer Chinese medicine —— Experimental research and clinical verification>> The book table or contents or directory (omitted)*

__*Volume IV*__ *<<To build the multidisciplinary and the science base of cancer-related research for conquering cancer- the Science City>> Contents (omitted)*

__*Volume V*__ *<<Theoretical Innovation of Cancer Prevention and Management or treatment cancer in the 21ˢᵗ Century>> Contents (Omitted)*

__*Volume VI*__ *<<XZ-C proposes to create the preventing cancer research institute and to carry out a series of cancer prevention projects>> Contents (Omitted)*

Dawning C plan
Dawning A·B·D plan
Prevention of Cancer and Treatment of Cancer and Preventin of Cancer and anti-cancer
The Dawning Science Research Program
The Dawning Scientific research spirit
Doctor is benevolence, to set up the moral is first

<u>Volume VII</u> <<Condense Wisdom and Conquer Cancer - Benefiting Mankind>> Contents (Omitted) (Volume I and II, which book has two parts)

<u>Volume VIII</u> <<The Road to Overcome Cancer>> Directory (omitted)

<u>Volume IX</u> <<On Innovation of Treatment of Cancer>> Contents (omitted)

<u>Volume X</u> <<New understanding and new models of cancer treatment>> Contents (omitted)

<u>Volume XI</u> <<New Concepts and New Methods for Cancer Metastasis Treatment>> Table of Contents (omitted)

<u>Volume XII</u> <<New Progress in Cancer Therapy>> Table of Contents (omitted)

<u>Volume XIII</u> <<New Concepts and New Methods for Cancer Treatment>> Table of Contents (omitted)

[Note: Each volume is a published monograph on cancer medical research]

<u>Note:</u>

1. *<u>XZ-C is Xu Ze-China, because science is borderless, but scientists have national and intellectual property.</u>*
2. *<u>Cancer is a disaster for all mankind. It must evoke the struggle of the people all over the world. Therefore, there are 8 monographs in the series, which are all in English, distributed worldwide, and published on **authorhouse.com**.</u>*

How to overcome cancer? How to prevent cancer? How to treat cancer? How to overcome cancer and to launch the general attack of cancer?

2.Professor Xu Ze (XZ-C) summed up the collection, agglutinated wisdom, and proposed 1 to 8 of "walk out of a new path to overcome cancer" in order to help or to facilitate clinical application and to become the clinical reference.

In the past 60 years, the series of the scientific research achievements and the series of scientific and technological innovations which takes "conquer cancer" as the direction done by us are in this series of "Monographs"; the following thesis or lemma are first proposed internationally, all of which are original papers, internationally pioneered, and have reached the forefront of the world.

XZ-C 's scientific thinking, scientific research design, academic thinking, and scientific dedication about conquering cancer and launching the total cancer attack are summarized as the following monographs:

1. "Walk out of a new road to conquer cancer" (1)(一)
   "Conquer cancer and launch the total attack to cancer – the prevention of cancer and cancer control and cancer treatment at the same level"

2. "Walk out of a new road to conquer cancer" (2) （二）
   "Walking out of a new way of cancer treatment with immune control and regulation of the combination of Chinese and Western medicine"
   (Part I), (Part 2)

3. "Walk out of a new road to conquer cancer" (3) （三）
   "The research of XZ-C immunomodulation anticancer Chinese medicine"
   — —Experimental research and clinical verification

4. "Walked out of a new road to conquer cancer" (4)(四)
**"Creating a Science City of Scientific Research Bases with Cancer Multidisciplinary and Cancer related research
For conquering cancer"**

5. "Walked out of a new road to conquer cancer" (5)(五)
"The Clinical Application Theory Innovation of 21ˢᵗ Century Cancer Prevention and Treatment Research"

6. "Walked out of a new road to conquer cancer" (6)(六)
XZ-C proposes <<to create the Cancer Prevention Research Institute of Environmental Protection >> and to carry out the system engineering of the cancer prevention

   (1). Prevention of Pollution and Treatment and Control of Pollution and Prevention of cancer and Anti-cancer anti-cancer
   (2). Dawning prevention cancer research plan and Dawning scientific research spirit
   (3). Medical is benevolence and set up the moral is the first

7. "Walk out of a new road to conquer cancer" (7) (七)
"Condense wisdom and conquer cancer - for the benefit of mankind" (part 1), (part 2)

8. "Walk out of a new road to conquer cancer" (8)(八)
"The Road to overcome cancer"

3. The monographs on cancer research published by Professor Xu Ze (XZ-C)

Professor Xu Ze continues to do the research after he retired, and the science's journey was non-stop, continues to achieve the following series of scientific research results.

In 1996, I was 63 years old and retired. After I retired, I have been living in a small building for more than 20 years. I have been working alone and fighting alone. I have continued a series of experimental studies and clinical verification observations. I have achieved the following series of scientific research results. The following monographs have been published.

Three monographs in Chinese version were published and distributed in the domestic nation

Twelve monographs in English version were published and distributed in the international.

**These 15 monographs are our hard journey, hard climbing, step by step, four different scientific research stages, four different levels of mountain results.**

1. Xu Ze etc (the first monograph published in the 67-year-old flower year) _"New understanding and new model of cancer treatment"_ Hubei Science and Technology Press, January 2001

2. Xu Ze etc (the second monograph published in the 73-year-old ancient rare year) _"New concept and new method of cancer metastasis treatment"_ published by Beijing People's Military Medical Press, January 2006; "Three One hundred original book certificate" was issued by the People's Republic of China Publishing House in April 2007

3. Xu Ze etc (the third book published in the 78-year-old ancient year) *"New concept and new method of cancer treatment"* published by Beijing People's Military Medical Press, October 2011; later the American medical doctor Dr. Bin Wu translated into English, the English edition was published in Washington, DC on March 26, 2013.

4. Xu Ze etc (the third edition of the special edition of the English version was published in the 80-year-old year) *"New Concept and New Way Of Treatment of Cancer"*, published in USA in March 2013 in English, internationally distributed

5. Xu Ze etc (the fifth book published at the age of 82) **"On Innovation of Treatment of Cancer"**, published in USA in December 2015, full English version, global distribution

6. Xu Ze etc (published the sixth monograph at the age of 83) **"New Concept and New Way of Treatment of Cancer Metastais"** published on August 2016 in USA in English, global issued

7. Xu Ze etc (the seventh book was published at the age of 83) **"The Road To Over Come Cancer"**, published in USA in December 2016 in English, published worldwide.

8. Xu Ze etc (published the eighth monograph at the age of 86) **"Condense Wisdom and Conquer Cancer for the Benefit of Mankind"**

Volume I: How to overcome cancer? How to prevent cancer? In December 2017

Published in USA in English and distributed globly

Volume II: How to overcome cancer? How to treat cancer? In February 2018

9. Xu Ze etc (the ninth monograph was published in the year of 87) **"The New progress in Cancer Treatment"**, published in USA in June 2018 in English, globally distributed

10. Xu Ze etc (the eleventh monograph was published in the year of 87 years old) *"Conquer Cancer and Launch The Total attack to Cancer"* in USA in November 2018 Published, full English, global distribution(Volume I)

11. Xu Ze etc(the twelfth monograph was published in the year of 88 years old) **"Walked Out of the New Road to Conquer Cancer" (part I) (Volume II)** in USA in January 2019 published, full English, global distribution

Walked Out of the New Way of Cancer Treatment with Immune Regulation and Control of Combination of Chinese and Western Medicine

12. Xu Ze etc(the thirteenth monograph was published in the year of 88 years old) **Walked Out of the New Road to Conquer Cancer(part II)**(Volume III) in USA in January 2019 published, full English, global distribution

Walked Out of the New Way of Cancer Treatment with Immune Regulation and Control of the Combination of Chinese and Western Medicine

13. Xu Ze etc(the fourteenth monograph was published in the year of 88 years old) **The Research on Anticancer Traditional Chinese Medication with Immune Regulation and Control** (Volume IV) in USA in February 2019 published, full English, global distribution ——Experimental Research and Clinical Application Verification

14. Xu Ze etc(the fifteenth monograph was published in the year of 88 years old) **Innovation on Clinical Application Theory of Cancer Prevention and Treatment Research in the 21st Century**

(Volume V) in USA in February 2019 published, full English, global distribution

GUIDANCE

How to overcome cancer, how to prevent cancer by I see
How can I treat cancer by I see

XZ-C found problems and raised problems from the follow-up results (Hint: how to prevent postoperative recurrence and metastasis is the key to improve long-term outcomes after surgery)

↓

Pathfinding (to overcome cancer, where is the road? How do you find it?)

↓

Pathfinding and footprint (the series of the scientific research results and scientific and technological innovation of cancer prevention and anti-cancer metastasis research)

↓

Published cancer monographs (3 Chinese editions are exclusively distributed nationwide, 5 full English editions are published worldwide)

↓

Participated in the International Congress of Oncology (AACR Academic Conference in USA)

↓

Visiting the Stirling Cancer Institute in Houston, USA (2009)

↓

Accumulated Basic and clinical research on prevention of cancer and anti-cancer metastasis in the past more than 60 years

↓

Accumulated the clinical application experience from more than 12,000 cases in the past more than 34 years

↓

<u>Walked Out of a new road to treat cancer with an immune regulatory and control of the combination of Chinese and Western medicine at the molecular level</u>

↓

1. *Walking out of a new road of cancer treatment to conquer cancer, "Chinese-style anti-cancer", Chinese and Western medicine combined with immune regulation and control*

2. *Published the English monograph "The Road to Overcome Cancer" in December 6, 2016, published in USA global distribution by Author house press, INC*

3. *Published the English monograph "Condense Wisdom and Conquer Cancer" in December 2017 (Volume I), published in February 2018 (Volume II) in USA, full English version, global distribution by Author house press, Inc*

4. *Published the English monograph "Conquer Cancer and launch The Total Attack to Cancer" – cancer prevention and cancer control and cancer treatment at the same level and at the same attention published in November 2018(Volume I) in the United States by Authorhouse.com, global distribution*

5. *Xu Ze etc (the ninth monograph was published in the year of 87) "The New progress in Cancer Treatment", published in USA in June 2018 in English, globally distributed*

6. *Xu Ze etc (the eleventh monograph was published in the year of 87 years old) "Conquer Cancer and Launch The Total attack to Cancer" in USA in November 2018 Published, full English, global distribution(Volume I)*

7. *Xu Ze etc(the twelfth monograph was published in the year of 88 years old) "Walked Out of the New Road to Conquer Cancer" (part I) (Volume II) in USA in January 2019 published, full English, global distribution*
Walked Out of the New Way of Cancer Treatment with Immune Regulation and Control of Combination of Chinese and Western Medicine

8. *Xu Ze etc(the thirteenth monograph was published in the year of 88 years old) Walked Out of the New Road to Conquer Cancer(part II)(Volume III) in USA in January 2019 published, full English, global distribution*
Walked Out of the New Way of Cancer Treatment with Immune Regulation and Control of the Combination of Chinese and Western Medicine

9. *Xu Ze etc(the fourteenth monograph was published in the year of 88 years old) The Research on Anticancer Traditional Chinese Medication with Immune Regulation and Control (Volume IV) in USA in February 2019 published, full English, global distribution ——Experimental Research and Clinical Application Verification*

10. *Xu Ze etc(the fifteenth monograph was published in the year of 88 years old)* *Innovation on Clinical Application Theory of Cancer Prevention and Treatment Research in the 21ᵗʰ Century*
(Volume V) in USA in February 2019 published, full English, global distribution

11. *Xu Ze etc (the fifth book published at the age of 82)* *"On Innovation of Treatment of Cancer", published in USA in December 2015, full English version, global distribution*

ACKNOWLEDGEMENTS

This book is for all of people who concern human being health. We are deeply grateful to all of people who like our new ways to improve our human being health.

I appreciated all of the people who encourage us to finish all of these books. Life is extremely difficult some time, *for example in the evening in Winter it was extremely cold of sticking into my bone in my room while these book were finished. Many times I woke up by this cold.*

I pray and pray for God's support. Challenges! I am a brave solider to prevent others.

My daughter **Lily Xu** gave me many smart and creative ideas while we were finishing this book and she is really bright light for my life and gives me encouragement such as during the cold weather she came to all of the dance and music and other classes after the regular school and during the weekend to get extra study. Lily Xu drew all of the pictures such as the Thymus and cancer stages and cancer metastasis steps and stages etc. **The characteristics of she loves the challenge** and **her judgment always encourages me to continue working hard to move on**.

I would like to express our sincere gratitude to the following:

1. All of Authorhouse staffs
2. All of the persons who encourage me.

Bin Wu, M.D., Ph.D

03-08-2018 in Baltimore, Maryland in USA

Prevention Cancer ● Anti-Cancer

Conquer Cancer ● Launch the General Attack

Condense Wisdom ● Conquer Cancer

FOREWORD(1)

This book is used to conquer cancer and launch the general attack on cancer and to create the Science City for conquering cancer. XZ-C's overall design, planning, and blueprint of the scientific research projects for conquering cancer is the scientific thinking and theoretical innovation and experimental basis for conquering cancer. It is the overall strategic reform and development of cancer treatment in China. It is **my 60 years of experience in medical work** and **30 years of scientific research results** and **the scientific and technological innovation and the scientific thinking and scientific research wisdom** which conquering cancer is as the research direction. Now It is planned to set up a test area in the Huangjiahu University City of Wuhan City. The research project will be implemented by experts and professors of the research team.

The scientific research plan of conquering cancer is a key scientific research in the world and is the frontier of science.

On January 12, 2016, US President Barack Obama proposed the National Cancer Program "Conquering Cancer" in his State of the Union address, and named the Cancer Moon Shot, which was implemented by Vice President Biden. The specific plan is unknown.

Cancer is a disaster for all mankind. It must fight globally. The people of the world should work together to gather wisdom and to advance together to overcome cancer.

The disaster of cancer covers the whole world. People all over the world are eager to hope to overcome cancer one day. It is hoped that the state, government, experts, scholars and scientists can find out prevention cancer measures to keep people away from cancer.

FOREWORD(2)

Overview

I am a retired medical professor. I am 86 years old and I am a white-haired old man. It is already the year of wind candle and years of ruin. I like to read the "Government Work Report" proposed in 2018... speed up the construction of innovative countries; ...... Strengthen research on smog or pollution control and promote the prevention and treatment of major diseases such as cancer; make technology better for the benefit of the people; ......resolutely fight the three major battles; ... anti-fouling or pollution prevention and pollution control. This makes me ecstatic. This is the current generation, benefiting the future, seeking health and welfare for the people which it is a great move for the health and welfare of future generations.

President Xi said: *"People's longing for a better life is the goal of our struggle. "*Cancer disasters cover the whole world, the current cancer incidence is increasing, and the cancer mortality rate is high. The people of the whole country and the people all over the world are eagerly looking forward to one day to overcome cancer. It is hoped that the state, government, experts and scholars will find out anti-cancer measures so that people can stay away from cancer.

Now we are delighted with the prosperity of our country, the spring of science, and the innovation of science and technology. Under the guidance of President Xi's new era of socialism with Chinese characteristics, in this new era, the new journey, the scientific research work to overcome the prevention and treatment of cancer should be advanced. In the "Nineteenth National Congress" of the Party and the work report of the current NPC government, it has clearly stated that it is necessary to treat smog and conquer cancer as the two major scientific and technological issues of the country. In the "Government Work Report", we have issued a great call to strengthen the management of smog and promote cancer prevention and control to benefit the people. Our medical workers and science and technology workers should respond and resolutely implement them. I will try my best to contribute this scientific research to the motherland and to the people of the motherland. *Although I am the age of 86 years old, the old man, in this new era of science spring, it is still motivating me to work hard to advance scientific research efforts to overcome cancer. The old man knows that his time is short and he does not need to raise his own whip.*

Because in the past 30 years, I have made a series of basic research and clinical observation research on anti-cancer and anti-metastasis research which is taking "conquer cancer " as the research direction and has achieved a series of scientific research results and technological innovation series or a series of scientific research achievements and technological innovation series have been obtained.

I want to resolutely implement the "Government Work Report" on prevention pollution and pollution control; ... Strengthening research on haze management; ... to advance research on prevention and treatment of major cancer diseases, make technology better for the benefit of the people; ... Resolutely fight the three major battles... prevention pollution and pollution control and pollution treatment . I will dedicate my scientific thinking, scientific thinking. For 30 years, I have taken scientific wisdom of which have been taking "conquer cancer " as the research direction, contribute to my motherland and our province and the people of our city. Now summarize how to promote cancer prevention and treatment research? how to overcome cancer? how to prevent cancer? and how to conquer cancer? how to treat cancer? how to scientifically prevent pollution and pollution to achieve the effect of first-class prevention cancer and anti-cancer, the following is an overview or make the following overview.

1. In view of the increasing incidence of cancer, the more patients are treated, the more patients; the cancer mortality rate is still staying high or remains high, how to change this current situation?

We believe that: It is imperative to change the current mode of running the hospital with attention of treatment and light protection or only treatment of cancer without prevention into **the mode of prevention and treatment at the same level and at the same attention**, so as to reduce cancer incidence, reduce cancer death, improve cancer cure rate, and prolong survival. It is recommended to carry out "to conquer cancer and to launch a general attack - prevention, control, and treatment of cancer at the same level and at the same attention."

After 30 years of cancer research and clinical research which have been taking "conquer cancer" as the direction, **we deeply understand that we want to achieve the prevention of cancer and anti-cancer and cancer control purposes**.

1). The general attack must be launched, that is, **the three stages of prevention of cancer, cancer control, and cancer treatment are equally important.** The three carriages go hand in hand to reduce the incidence of cancer, improve the cure rate of cancer, reduce cancer mortality, and prolong the survival of patients.

If it is only to treat cancer without prevention of cancer, or attention to treatment with light defense and paid more attention to treatment only, it is never possible to overcome cancer because it does not reduce the incidence of cancer, and the more patients are treated and the more patient.

The current mode of running a hospital should be changed, from only attention to treatment and light prevention into prevention of cancer and cancer control and treatment cancer at the same level and at the same attention and at the same time.

It should change the current treatment mode, *from the treatment of serious illness in the advanced stage and only the emphasis on the middle and late stages of treatment into more emphasis on "three early", (early detection, early diagnosis, early treatment), precancerous lesions, early carcinoma in situ.*

This will benefit mankind and will open up a new era of anti-cancer research, making China's cancer prevention and treatment industry into the forefront of the world.

How to launch a general attack? To implement cancer prevention + cancer control + cancer treatment, it is necessary to establish the hospital which is paying attention to prevention and treatment and control of cancer during the occurrence and development, and to reform the current mode of running the hospital of treatment only without prevention, and to reform the current treatment mode of the middle or advanced stage cancer. Therefore, our proposal puts forward: to carry out the report *"To conquer cancer and launch the general attack of cancer; the prevention, control, and treatment at the same time and at the same level and at the same attention."* This is an unprecedented event, reported to the Party Central Committee and the State Council, and applied for leadership, support, implementation, and implementation by the leaders of the Hubei Provincial Party Committee and the provincial government.

2). In order to carry out prevention of cancer and cancer control work, the government leadership, leadership, experts and scholars must work hard, the masses should participate, and thousands of households can participate. At present, China is building an innovative country. It is the government-led, the masses' participation, and the work of thousands of households. This is a good time. If you can carry out medical scientific research to overcome cancer, cancer prevention, and cancer control, it will definitely improve the awareness of cancer prevention among the people and achieve the effect of preventing cancer and controlling cancer and receive that effect of significantly reduce the incidence of cancer in China, in the providence and in the city.

3). I have been conducting basic research and clinical validation for cancer research for 30 years as the direction of conquering cancer, both in laboratories and hospitals. Why do I need to apply for government support now?

Because 90% of cancers are related to the environment, the occurrence of cancer is closely related to people's clothing, food, housing, travel and lifestyle. Therefore, I deeply think that prevention cancer and cancer control work can not be done by medical personnel, experts and scholars alone. It must rely on the government's major policies. The current environmental pollution is serious and the ecosystem is degraded, which may be closely related to the rising incidence of cancer.

The treatment of cancer currently relies on medical personnel and researchers to research new drugs and new treatment technologies.

However cancer prevention and control, how to reduce the incidence of cancer, cancer prevention work must rely on the government's major policy, relying on government leadership and leadership, experts and scholars to work hard, the masses can participate.

2. It is given the complexity of oncology, the etiology, pathogenesis, pathophysiology, and biological behavior of cancer cells ? Metastasis mechanism? Why do cancer cells fall off? Why can there be implantation or metastasis or recurrence mechanism? A series of oncology and tumor related issues are not well understood. Oncology is still a scientific virgin land for scientific research. A lot of basic science and clinical basic research are needed. To conduct basic research in cancer science, it is an urgent need of the current oncology discipline.

It is necessary to establish a group of specialist research groups closely related to cancer, specializing in molecular level basic and clinical research, in order to find related anti-cancer, cancer treatment theories, techniques, drugs, methods and measures. Set up while developing.

1). In 2013-2014-2015 I have been researching and developing basic ideas and designs for how to overcome cancer; Formulate the theoretical basis and experimental basis for how to overcome cancer;

Formulate the guidelines, methods of planning, and blue figure of how to conquer cancer, then came up with:

a. *"XZ-C research plan of conquering cancer and launching the general attack of cancer"*

b. *"Report on the Necessity of Preparing for the Prevention and Treatment of Cancer in the Whole Process"*

c. *The general Planning and general design of "Building a Scientific Research Base for conquering cancer and launching the General Attack of Cancer and Multi-disciplinary and Cancer-Related Research-----the scientific city"*

<u>*This research project was first proposed internationally, opening up new areas of anti-cancer research.*</u>

XZ-C proposed to overcome cancer and launch the general attack of cancer, which is unprecedented work. How to conquer cancer, this is the world's leading science front and science - there is no end to the front. *Leaders, experts, scholars, and entrepreneurs should be invited to participate in practice, implementation, and implementation.*

2). From July 2015, we formulated the "Dawning C-type plan", that is, dawn is morning light, Chaoyang, C type = China, that is, "China style modelmodel", a plan of conquering cancer

How to overcome cancer? How to treat cancer?

XZ-C proposes: Dawning C-type plan No. 1 - 6

Dawning C-type plan No. 1: "Overcoming cancer and launching the general attack of cancer"
Dawning C-type plan No. 2: "Creating a full-scale prevention or defense and treatment hospital"
Dawning C-type plan No. 3: "Building a science city to overcome cancer"
Dawning Type C Plan No. 4: "Building a Multidisciplinary and Cancer Research Group"

Dawning C-type plan No. 5: "The vaccine is human hope, mmunological prevention"
Dawning Type C Plan No. 6:

A. *"The prospect of immunomodulatory drugs is gratifying"*
B. *"XZ-C immunomodulation of active ingredients of traditional Chinese medicine, establishment of molecular level research groups and laboratories"*

Therefore, we made a statement and proposed:

In order to conquer cancer, we should establish a scientific research base called "Science City for multidisciplinary and cancer-related research to overcome the general attack on cancer." ; to implement, realize Dawning C type 1-6.

3). How to overcome cancer? How to prevent cancer?

XZ-C proposes:

Create "the Innovative Environmental Protection and Prevention Cancer Research Institute" and carry out prevention cancer system engineering

XZ-C proposes:

Dawning A type anti-cancer plan

Dawning B type anti-cancer plan

Dawning D-type anti-cancer plan

How to implement this research plan of conquering cancer?

I detailed the general design and the master plan and the specific plan and program and blue map.

4). ***How to resolutely fight or win the battle of preventin pollution controlling pollution and treatment of smog or pollution?***

First, how about the three major sources of pollution? What is the source and formation of smog? It must find the bottom, conduct scientific analysis and scientific research. Where is the source? What are the consequences?

a. How does it produce and cause air pollution? Why lead to water pollution? Why does it cause soil pollution? What is the source? What are the consequences? How to solve?

What is the "target" of its research?

The research institutes of prevention of pollution and treatment pollution and pollution control should be established to conduct scientific research and experimental research.

b. What is pollution? What is the content of the pollution? What is the damage to human health?

Prevention of pollution or treatment of pollution and pollutant composition analysis rooms should be established.

Macroscopic, microscopic, ultra-microscopic

Equipment conditions: trace element analyzers, chemical analyzers... must establish state-level advanced laboratories, and our research team invites the Department of Chemistry of Wuhan University to cooperate to train graduate students to participate in practice.

Find out where the source of pollution is?

It should stop at the source, try to stop, ringing the bell and still need to ring the bell.

What is the content of pollution?

Microscopic, ultra-micro and biochemical, molecular biology, genetic engineering research and analysis should be carried out.

c. Establish pollutant detection and monitoring

It is implemented by the prevention of pollution or treatment pollution laboratory, and the monitoring report should be given.

d, The prevention of pollution and treatment pollution and the prevention of cancer and treatment cancer, cancer control research should be combined together to study and to do research

Where should the three targets of conquering pollution be targeted? How to solve?

e. XZ-C proposed to establish the "Innovative Environmental Protection and Health Prevention Cancer Research Institute" to carry out prevention cancer system engineering, and establish a high-level laboratory.

The party's 19ᵗʰ National Congress decided to resolutely fight and win the fight against or prevention pollution and controlling pollution, fighting hard, and strengthen research on smog governance. This is a great wise decision. Where did the three major pollution come from? XZ-C believes that this is a complication and sequelae in the development of human science and industrial production. These complications or sequelae must be carefully studied and cleared to stop it in order to improve the scientific development of modern times.

This is a wise and great move to improve the development of modern science, safeguard the human living environment, defend the human living environment, and defend human health.

These modern scientific developments have brought a beautiful life and living environment to human beings. But it also brings some negative complications and the negative effects of sequelae, affecting the living environment of human beings, the living environment, affecting human health, caused some cancerous changes, mutations, distortions because 90% of cancers are caused by environmental factors. Environmental factors lead to genetic mutations that lead to chromosomal deletions and abnormalities. Environmental factors can be managed and sought to find solutions. A newly published monograph "Gathering Wisdom, Conquering Cancer - Benefiting Mankind" is a medical monograph that is more comprehensive in design and specific planning for how to overcome cancer and is the outline for how to overcome cancer. This scientific research plan, scientific research plan, blue maps can be used for reference in various countries.

How to reduce or avoid these developmental complications and sequelae?

We should vigorously develop and <u>apply solar energy, water energy and wind energy as energy sources</u>. These come from natural sources of energy, such as collecting and storing well, then the complications after use, there will be little or no sequelae.

5). Analysis of the next research prospects

In short, modern medicine comes from Europe and the United States.

The development of modern medicine in the past 100 years has developed to microscopic → ultra-micro → precision medical nanotechnology, Chinese modern medicine relies heavily on imported drugs for cancer treatment. His own inventions, creations, patents, and intellectual property rights are small.

However the China advantages are:

1. Traditional Chinese medicine, anti-cancer traditional Chinese medicine, immune regulation traditional Chinese medicine, the traditional Chinese medicine with increasing blood circulation and removing the blood stasis and anti-cancer thrombosis, heat-clearing and detoxifying to improve cancer cells micro-environmental Chinese medicine, soft-firming and phlegm Chinese medicine with treatment of small knot cancer.

2. Combination of Chinese and Western medicine, combined with innovation.

The US advantage is:

Modernized medicine, advanced diagnosis and treatment technology, and targeted medicine.

We should give full play to China's advantages and potentials, and we should vigorously develop and explore the advantages of Chinese herbal medicine.

Our oncology lacks innovative medicine, medication, technology, innovative academics, theories, patents, and inventions of our own oncology. It must be self-reliant, independent innovation, original innovation, and achieve breakthrough medical and scientific achievements, then you will have your own medicine, medication, and scientific research results and you can have your own medicine, medication, and scientific and technological achievements which can compete and race with others.

Innovation is not only technology, product innovation, ***but also basic theoretical innovation, theoretical innovation is the biggest achievement. Scientific development is based on the innovation of basic theory, which is the biggest invention and creation.***

a. *We should give play to our advantages in areas where our country has advantages.* ***In the field of cancer research, traditional Chinese medicine is an advantage of China.*** ***We should make use of this advantage in cancer research to discover and develop effective Chinese herbal medicines for preventing cancer and cancer. We should*** *conduct in-depth research, conduct effective ingredient analysis and purification, conduct immunopharmacological research, conduct molecular and genetic level research, and make Chinese herbal medicines. The key to modernization and international integration is to establish a good laboratory.*

b. **The combination of Chinese and Western medicine is the characteristics and advantages of Chinese medicine. It comes from Chinese medicine,** *higher than Chinese medicine, it comes from Western medicine, higher than Western medicine, it is Chinese medicine + western medicine, 1+1=2, 2>1,* **which makes the treatment of cancer combined with Chinese and Western medicine more perfect and reasonable, and** improves the curative effect, extend patient survival, improve patient quality of life, and the standard of efficacy of evaluating cancer patients:

It should be that **the patient has lived for a long time (significantly prolonged survival), the quality of life is good, and the complications are no less or less.**

c. *Regardless of the complexity of the mechanisms behind cancer,* **immune suppression is the key to cancer progression.** *Removing the immunosuppressive factor and restoring the immune system's recognition of cancer cells can effectively prevent cancer. There is growing evidence that* **by regulating the body's immune system, it is possible to achieve cancer control.** *The treatment of tumors by activating the body's anti-tumor immune system is currently an area of interest for researchers. An important breakthrough in the next cancer is likely to come from this.*

d. Why do we look for drugs that promote thymic hyperplasia, prevent thymus atrophy, and boost immunity from traditional Chinese medicine?

Because Chinese medicine's tonic drugs generally contain the role of regulating immunity.

*Rehabilitation Chinese medicine or supporting Chinese medicine has the function of regulating immune function, and shows the dose-***effectiveness correlation under normal experimental conditions.**

When the animal is in low immunity (such as dethymus, aging animals, chemotherapeutic drugs cyclophosphamide inhibits immunization of animals), the tonic drugs improve the body's immunity is more significant.

Research on anti-cancer immunity of traditional Chinese medicine polysaccharides is progressing rapidly. A large number of immunopharmacological studies have been conducted at the molecular level. Most of them can improve the body's immune surveillance system and achieve the purpose of killing tumor cells. A large number of Chinese medicines have the effect of regulating the body's immune function.

e. *Our laboratory spent 4 years exploring the mechanism and regularity of <u>cancer metastasis</u> and looking for effective methods for anti-cancer metastasis; It took another three years to screen the animal experiments from 200 traditional Chinese herbal medicines through a rigorous scientific cancer-bearing animal model. The Results are that 48 kinds of XZ-C immunosuppressive anti-cancer and anti-metastatic traditional Chinese medicines with good tumor inhibition rate were screened out, then applied to the clinic based on this experimental study, the oncology clinic has more than 12,000 patients with advanced cancer in 30 <u>years, and has achieved good curative effect. It can prolong survival and improve the quality of life. From clinical to experimental, from experimental to clinical, basic and clinical integration is carried out. The combination of Chinese and Western medicines has brought out a new anti-cancer and anti-metastatic road with Chinese characteristics.</u>*

6). The above clarifies the basic and clinical research work that I have taken in the past 30 years to overcome cancer:

a). <u>*What research work have I done?*</u>

b). <u>*What research work are I doing?*</u>

c). <u>*What is my next step?*</u>

d). <u>*This work is significant, is an unprecedented work, we should go our own way.*</u>

Some people have, we must learn, we must have, Chinese herbal medication is the essence of Chinese culture. Efforts should be made to find out and improve, carry out active ingredient analysis, and conduct immunopharmacological analysis. In the field of cancer research, traditional Chinese medicine is an advantage of China. We should give full play to China's advantages and potentials, and we should vigorously develop and give full play to the advantages of Chinese herbal medicines, conduct molecular and genetic level studies and bring modernization of Chinese medicine into line with international standards, and to reach the world's pre-existence or precedent, the introduction of the combination of China and the West, the ancient is used for the present, the foreign is used in China, it is Chinese wisdom or, is the wisdom of China; the standard of the Evaluation of therapy efficacy of cancer:

It should be that the patient lives long, the quality of life is good, and the complications are no or little.

7). What should I do next? Now it is proposed to overcome cancer, launch a general attack, and hope to get support from leaders at all levels. I am deeply aware that in order to achieve the goal of cancer prevention, control, and treatment, it must be done by government leaders, government-led, experts and scholars, and the participation of the masses.

About 8550 people in China are diagnosed with cancer every day, and 6 people are diagnosed with cancer every minute. Therefore, research to overcome the scientific research work of cancer attack, can not walk slowly, should run forward, save the wounded.

No matter how far the road to conquer cancer is, you should always start, you should avoid talking, work hard, and start.

How to implement, how to achieve it, and hope to get the leading, leading and support of the provincial and municipal governments, I will do my best to participate in the implementation and implementation.

3. In the past 30 years, I have obtained a series of scientific research achievements and scientific and technological innovation series of anti-cancer and anti-cancer metastasis research. In the research work and the research work that has been carried out, it can be summarized into four major contributions to the people.

(1) For the first time in the world it is proposed that "to overcome cancer and to launch a general attack"

-----Changed the mode of running a hospital;

Changed treatment mode;

it is proposed the general attack design, blueprint and implementation rules and plans.

(2) The first proposed internationally

"Building a Science City of Conquering Cancer"

    ---- established an overall framework for the fight against cancer,

    This is the only way to overcome cancer;

    Proposed the overall design, blueprint and implementation rules. and plans of Science City

(3) First proposed internationally

"Walked out of the new way of overcoming cancer"

The experimental research, anti-cancer research with Chinese medicine immunopharmacology and molecular level Chinese and Western medicine combined

1). From the results of our laboratory experiments it is found:

After the host is inoculated with cancer cells, the host's thymus, that is, has acute progressive atrophy, cell proliferation is blocked, and the volume is significantly reduced.

2). From the above experimental research findings and the inspiration:

Thymus atrophy and low immune function may be one of the causes and pathogenesis of cancer. Therefore, tumor treatment must try to prevent thymus atrophy, promote thymocyte proliferation, and increase immunity.

3). After 7 years of scientific research in the laboratory, *we have screened XZ-C$_{1-10}$ immunomodulatory anti-cancer and anti-metastatic Chinese medicine from natural medicine, and carried out clinical verification work based on the success of animal experiments. More than 12,000 clinical applications in 20 years of oncology clinics have achieved good results.*

4). Walked out with a traditional Chinese medicine immune regulation, regulate immune activity, prevent thymus atrophy, promote thymic hyperplasia, protect bone marrow hematopoietic function, improve immunity, and combine Western medicine with new water to overcome cancer.

5). We have embarked on an XZ-C immune regulation, and the combination of Chinese and Western medicine at the molecular level has overcome the road to cancer

6). "Chinese-style anti-cancer" new road.

(4) Exclusive research and development XZ-C immune regulation anti-cancer Chinese medicine series products

——Experimental research+clinical application+typical case+case list

—— XZ-C (XU ZE-China) (Xu Ze-China), an independently developed anti-cancer series of traditional Chinese medicine preparations, from experimental research to clinical verification, applied to clinical practice on the basis of successful animal experiments. After more than 12,000 clinical trials in more than 20 years, the curative effect is remarkable, and it is independent innovation and independent intellectual property rights.

——XZ-C immunomodulatory Chinese medicine, from the more than 200 traditional Chinese herbal medicines in China, 48 kinds of Chinese herbal medicines with good tumor inhibition rate were screened by anti-tumor experiments in cancer-bearing mice. After the compound is compounded, the tumor-inhibiting experiment is carried out in the cancer-bearing mice. The compound tumor inhibition rate is greater than that of single-flavor drug inhibition. Among them, XZ-C1 100% inhibits cancer cells, 100% does not kill normal cells, and has the function of strengthening the body and improving the immune function of the human body.

From our experiments on XZ-C pharmacodynamics studies:

It has a good tumor inhibition rate for Ehrlich ascites carcinoma, S180, H22 liver cancer. Acute toxicity test in mice showed no obvious side effects. In the clinical oral administration for several years (2-6-8-10 years), no obvious side effects were observed.

In the middle and late stage cancer patients, most of them are weak and weak, tired and weak, and their appetite is weak. After taking XZ-C immunomodulation anti-cancer Chinese medicine for 4-8-12 weeks, they can significantly improve appetite, sleep, relieve pain, and gradually recover the physical strength.

(5) At present, the country is implementing the spirit of the party's "Nineteenth National Congress", ensuring that a well-off society will be built nationwide in 2020, rejuvenating Greater China, building an innovative country, and resolutely fighting to win three major battles, anti-pollution, pollution control, and smog control and conquer cancer. This is a great pioneering work for the benefit of the country and the people. Under this great situation, it has also created good opportunities for the research work of preventing cancer, fighting cancer and conquering cancer. The purpose is to protect the people's health and stay away from cancer. It is also a great initiative for the health and welfare of future generations.

Do something big and do an unprecedented event, "To overcome conquer and launch the general attack of cancer," "Create a science city to overcome cancer," for the benefit of mankind.

How to implement this unprecedented event in human history?

It is suggested:

It is prepared in Hubei and Wuhan to build up:

"The first science city in the country to overcome cancer research base";

"The world's first science city to conquer cancer research base"

Site selection:

Plans to be in the university town of Huangjiahu;

Abbreviation: "Huangjiahu Science City" Cancer Medical Research Center;

It strive to build in 5 years up;

Started in 2019 and completed in 2023;

And it can serve cancer patients nationwide and globally.

4. It requires leadership support:

Conquering cancer and launching the general attack of cancer is an unprecedented work of humanity. It must be created in person and must be practiced in person. This is a new cement road that will leave an eternal scientific footprint every step of the way.

In the "Nineteenth National Congress" of the Party and the work report of the current NPC government, it has clearly stated that it is necessary to treat smog and conquer cancer as the two major scientific and technological issues of the country. To this end, our medical workers and science and technology workers must actively promote and have implementation.

I am convinced that under the leadership, guidance, support and care of the provincial and municipal leaders, with the efforts of my team, it will be completed as scheduled to benefit the majority of cancer patients.

The chief designer of "To overcome the general attack on cancer and to build a cancer research base - Science City" **and the Head of the discipline** of "Overcoming the general attack on cancer" and the **Honorary President** of Wuhan Anticancer Research Association and the **Former Director** of the Institute of Experimental Surgery and Hubei University of Traditional Chinese Medicine

↓

Professor Xu Ze

02-2019 In Wu Han, China

Walked out of the new road to conquer cancer 6 (六) (Vol. 6)

(The new concept of XZ-C cancer prevention and treatment)

Conquer cancer and Launch a general attack

<<Multidisciplinary and the research base of the Cancer Research Group for conquering cancer and launching the general attack to cancer – the Science City>>

The General Design, Blueprint and Preparation Work (1)

(Volume 1)

TABLE OF CONTENTS

Volume I

—

The Proposal for Cancer Treatment Reform and Innovation and Development

I have been engaged in the clinical work of oncology surgery for 60 years. In 1991, I suffered from acute myocardial infarction. After rescued, I recovered after half a year of hospitalization; I can not go on stage to do surgery, calm down, hide in the small building, concentrate on the basics and clinical aspects of cancer. After 28 years of hard work, a series of experimental research and clinical verification work were carried out, and a series of scientific and technological innovations were obtained.

I am a clinical surgeon, why do I study cancer? This is due to the results of a petition to a group of cancer patients after surgery.

In 1985, I conducted a petition to more than 3,000 patients operated by my own with postoperative chest and abdominal cancer. RESULTS: Most patients were found to have recurrence or metastasis 2 to 3 years after surgery, and some even relapsed and metastasized several months after surgery. From the results of the follow-up, we found:

Postoperative recurrence and metastasis are the key factors affecting the long-term efficacy of surgery. Therefore, it also raised an important question for us: that is, clinicians must pay attention to and study the prevention and treatment measures for postoperative recurrence and metastasis, so as to improve the long-term efficacy after operation. **Therefore, clinically based experimental studies must be conducted.**

So we established the Laboratory of Animal Experimental Surgery (the Institute of Experimental Surgery of Hubei College of Traditional Chinese Medicine was

1

established in 1991, and the research direction was to overcome cancer). We spent 20 years in the following three aspects and conducted a series of experimental studies and clinical validation work.

1. Conducted a series of experimental tumor studies:

Cancer cell transplantation was performed to establish a cancer-bearing animal model; it explored the mechanisms and rules of cancer pathogenesis, invasion, metastasis, and recurrence; and it searched the effective measures to regulate and control the cancer invasion, metastasis, and recurrence.

We have conducted a full 4 years of oncology research work in the laboratory, which is the topic of clinical basic research and the selections of the research projects all are clinically proposed to explain or solve these clinical problems through experimental research.

It was found from the experimental tumor research in our laboratory:

(1) Our laboratory removes the thymus from the mouse (30 Kunming mice), which can be used to produce a cancer-bearing animal model. Injection of immunosuppressive agents can also contribute to the establishment of a cancer-bearing animal model.

The research conclusions prove that:the occurrence and development of cancer are obviously related to the thymus and its function of the host immune organs.

(2) Whether it is low immunity first and then easy to get cancer, or cancer occurs first and then it has the low immunity?

The results of the experiment are*: first, there is low immunity and then cancer occurs and develops. If there is no immune function, it is not easy to be vaccinated successfully.*

The results of this experiment suggest:

Improving and maintaining good immune function is one of the important measures to prevent cancer.

(3) When we explore the effects of tumors on immune organs in the body, it was found that as the cancer progressed, the thymus was atrophied (600 mice bearing

cancer model mice), and the host thymus was acute progressive atrophy after inoculation of cancer cells.

(4) The above experimental results prove that:

The progression of the tumor can cause progressive atrophy of the thymus. *So, **can we use some methods to prevent the host's thymus atrophy?*** Therefore, we further design and want to look for ways or drugs to prevent thymic atrophy in tumor-bearing mice through animal experiment researches. Therefore, we used this immune organ cell transplantation to restore the experimental function of the immune organ. We are discussing "Stop the atrophy of the immune thymus during tumor progression", looking for ways to restore the function of the thymus and rebuild the immune system. The mice were used for fetal liver cells, fetal spleen cells, fetal thymocyte transplantation, and experimental studies on the immune function of adoptive immune reconstitution. The results show: S, T, L three groups of cells were transplanted together (200 experimental mice). The tumor regression rate was 40% in the near future, and the complete regression rate in the long-term tumor was 46.67%. The patients with complete tumor regression had long-term survival.

Based on the findings of the above experimental research, we present in the second chapter of the book "New Concepts and New Methods of Cancer Therapy": "Thymus atrophy and low immune function are one of the pathogenesis of cancer." In Chapter 3, the theoretical basis and experimental basis of "XZ-C immune regulation therapy for breast enhancement" are presented. It was reported at the International Oncology Society in Washington in September 2013, which attracted widespread attention and high attention.

2. The Experimental Study of looking for and screening new anticancer and anticancer drugs from traditional Chinese medicine

In our laboratory through In vivo anti-tumor experiments by animal models of cancer-bearing mice, searching for traditional Chinese medicines that inhibit cancer cells without affecting normal cells and traditional Chinese medicines that inhibit cancer cell metastasis was done. *We spent a full three years and the traditional Chinese herbal medicines used in traditional anti-cancer prescriptions and anti-cancer agents reported in various places were subjected to tumor-suppressing screening experiments in cancer-bearing animals.* The tumor-inhibiting screening experiment in cancer-bearing animals was carried out one by one. Through in vivo anti-tumor screening experiments on 200 traditional "anti-cancer Chinese medicine" cancer-bearing animal models, it was found that: Among them, 48 kinds of traditional Chinese medicines have inhibitory effects on cancer cells, and 26 kinds of traditional Chinese medicines have the effect of increasing immune regulation (excluding 152 kinds of cancer cells have no inhibitory effect).

After optimized combination, the tumor-inhibiting experiment in the animal model of cancer can be used to observe the effects of thymus, spleen, liver and kidney, and form $XZ-C_{1-10}$ anticancer traditional Chinese medicine preparation. $XZ-C_1$ can significantly inhibit cancer cells, but does not affect Normal cell, $XZ-C_4$ can promote thymic hyperplasia and increase immunity; $XZ-C_8$ protects the bone marrow from hematopoiesis. XZ-C immunomodulatory Chinese medicine can improve the quality of life of patients with advanced cancer, increase immunity, enhance the body's ability to fight cancer, enhance physical fitness, increase appetite, and significantly improve symptoms.

3. Clinical verification work

Through the above four years to explore the basic experimental research on recurrence and metastasis mechanisms and after three years of experimental research from natural Chinese herbal medicines, a batch of $XZ-C_{1-10}$ immunomodulatory cancer drugs was identified.

Then through Clinical validation of the oncology specialist outpatient clinic in 16 years, more than 12,000 cases in the middle and late stages or postoperative metastasis of cancer patients, application of XZ-C immunomodulation of anticancer Chinese medicine has achieved good results, and can improve the quality of life of patients, improve patient symptoms and significantly prolong patient survival.

4. Briefly describe the history of anti-cancer research

(1) After I have recovered my heart attack, I should take a good rest. Why did I conduct a series of basic and clinical research on cancer?

In April 1991, the author submitted an application for key scientific and technological projects to the State Science and Technology Commission.

The project name is "further explore the experimental and clinical research on the prevention and treatment of anti-cancer and anti-cancer Chinese herbal medicine for the prevention and treatment of precancerous lesions of gastric cancer, liver cancer and gastric cancer."

In June, Director of the Hubei Provincial Science and Technology Commission organized the heads of the three projects of the province to apply for the National Science and Technology Commission. (1 person from Tongji Medical College, 1 from Hubei Medical College and 1 from Hubei College of Traditional Chinese Medicine) went to Beijing to report to the Chinese Medicine Administration of the Ministry of Health. Two months later, Director Tian of the Provincial Science and Technology Commission and three project leaders went to Beijing to report further to the Ministry of Health on design and acceptance of the project. *Two months later, when the project task was issued and he was planning to sign a special contract for the national science and technology research project, Professor Xu Ze suddenly developed acute myocardial infarction, anterior wall and high wall myocardial infarction.*

After rescue and treatment, hospitalized for half a year, after leaving the hospital for half a year, I gradually recovered. The National Science and Technology Commission will also be stranded and suspended.

In 1993, Professor Xu Ze's physical health gradually recovered, and he also thought about continuing to study the content of the subject. Because the author has followed up the patients after high-cost radical resection, it turned out, postoperative recurrence and metastasis of cancer are the key factors affecting the long-term outcome after radical resection of cancer. The clinical basis and effective methods for preventing postoperative recurrence and metastasis must be studied.

It was determined to do some research work that should be done within this capacity. However there are only ideas but there is no research funding. So I began to find ways to raise funds for research.

In 1993, when the author's wife was retired, she applied for a clinic, and her meager income was the starting point for research funding. Kunming mice were purchased from the Animal Center of the Medical College for animal experiments, animal cages and related equipment and instruments were prepared, and animal experiments were started. The meager income of the clinic is used to support Professor Xu Ze's animal experiments and scientific research, and to save money in careful calculation. Six rooms on the second floor were used for animal experiments. *In 1996, Professor Xu Ze was 63 years old and applied for retirement. After that, with the support of this meager income, a series of experimental studies and clinical validation work were carried out. After 20 years of hard work, finally, I basically completed the research project of the State Science and Technology Commission and combined experimental*

<u>and clinical research data, data, and summaries. By 2011, three monographs have been published.</u>

(2) Some experiences

In the past, the author conducted scientific research work in medical colleges. With the guidance of superiors and colleagues, the laboratory has excellent conditions, and has undertaken the National Natural Science Foundation project, the National Science and Technology Commission, and the Provincial Science and Technology Commission, which has achieved two scientific research results; one is the domestic advanced level, one is the international advanced level, and won the second prize of Hubei Province Science and Technology Achievements twice, and won the first prize of Hubei Provincial Health Science and Technology Achievements. But now it is different. In this special case, in a clinic or clinic, under the condition of unconditional and no equipment, how can we carry out and complete national task tasks? The author has the following brief experience.

1. Self-reliance and self-financing. See the outpatient service for the patient service, and the outpatient income is used as research funding.

2. Keep outpatient medical records and follow up.

3. Establish special research collaborations, collaborate and cooperate according to scientific research plans.

4. to establish detailed medical records (including patient epidemiological data), in-depth analysis of each successful experience of treatment, the lessons of failure and the particularity of the condition.

5. With the scientific research cooperation strategy of instrument sharing, equipment sharing and results sharing, we will not add large-scale instruments and equipment. In collaboration with the Medical College Affiliated Hospital, high-precision instrumentation and equipment inspections were conducted in the Medical College Affiliated Hospital.

6. Self-selected scientific frontiers, failed to declare the subject (because it has been nearly ancient and rare); to be studied, only the research results will be reported to the Ministry, the province and the city.

7. The old professors in a private outpatient department, through the cooperation with universities and colleges scientific research collaboration and equipment, the strategy of sharing results; by making full use of the advanced equipment conditions of colleges and universities and combining decades of clinical experience, we can also carry out and complete research projects.

__After 20 years of hard work, a series of experimental research and clinical verification work were carried out. I finally basically completed the content of the "Eighth Five-Year Plan" project of the National Science and Technology Commission that I applied for__. The experimental and clinical research material or information, data, conclusions, summary collections, which were written more than one hundred scientific research papers. Since there is no research funding, they cannot be send magazines for publication so that it was published in accordance with the new books. Three monographs have been published successively.

5. Outline anti-cancer research and research results

(1) published monographs on cancer research

After 20 years of hard work and hard work, it was carried out a series of experimental research and clinical validation work, the experimental and clinical validation data collation which was my more than 50 years of clinical case review, analysis, reflection, experience and my own more than a decade of cancer experimental results and discoveries from the experimental to clinical, but also from clinical to experimental was summed up the collection and published as three monographs: 1, "new understanding of cancer treatment and new model", Hubei Science and Technology Publishing House, Xu Ze In January 2001. 2, "new concept and new methods of cancer metastasis ", published by the Beijing People's Medical Publishing House, Xu Ze, January 2006. In April 2007 issued by the People's Republic of China issued a "three hundred" original book certificate. 3, "new concepts and new methods of cancer treatment", published by the Beijing People's Medical Publishing House, Xu Ze / Xu Jie, October 2011. Followed by American physician Dr. Bin Wu translated into English. The English version was published in Washington on March 26, 2013 and was issued internationally.

These three monographs are our difficult trek, hard climbing, step by step in the three different scientific research stages of scientific research, three different levels of achievement. (**The first monograph at the age of 67, the second monograph at the age of 73, the third monograph at the age of 78, the English version of the**

third monograph at the age of 80, the English edition, the Washington issue, the international distribution)

(2) Brief description of anti-cancer, anti-cancer metastasis research results

We have 38 years (1985-----) cancer research work in animal experiments, clinical basic research, clinical validation work has made a series of scientific and technological innovation scientific and technological achievements. As the contents are more, here is only directory, research topics and belongs to the original innovation or independent innovation.

① **"thymus atrophy, immune dysfunction is one of the causes of cancer and pathogenesis"**

--The new discovery in the study of the etiology and pathogenesis of cancer was proposed or advanced

② **" The theoretical basis and experimental basis of protection of thymus and increasing immune function of XZ-C immunomodulation therapy"**

- -The theoretical basis and experimental basis of immunoregulation therapy for cancer were put forward

③ **"cancer treatment should change the concept and establish a comprehensive treatment concept"**

-- put forward the new concept of cancer treatment principles

④ **"The assembling new model of cancer multidisciplinary comprehensive treatment"**

⑤ **" the analysis, evaluation and questioning of solid tumor systemic intravenous chemotherapy"**

-- questioned the traditional drug administration approach, the dose calculation and the efficacy evaluation of the treatment of systemic cancer therapy for systemic intravenous chemotherapy

⑥ **" the initiative to change the solid body tumor intravenous chemotherapy into the target organ intravascular chemotherapy"**

- -Advocacy for changing traditional cancer therapy or

-- Initiative of reforming traditional cancer therapy

⑦ **"the initiative of the improvement measures on postoperative cancer adjuvant chemotherapy"**

-- Advocacy for reforming traditional cancer chemotherapy

⑧ **" there are three main existing forms of cancer in the human body"**

--Advice on the new concept of cancer metastasis therapy

--The third form is the group of cancer cells that are being metastasis on the way

⑨ The **"two points and one line " during the whole process of cancer development**

--Advice on the therapy innovation of cancer metastasis therapy

⑩ **" the three steps of anti-cancer treatment"**

- Propose the theoretical innovation of the new concept of cancer metastasis therapy

- The "eight steps" of the metastasis of cancer cells are summarized as "three stages" and try to break each step

⑪ **"open up the third field of anti-cancer metastasis therapy"**

----- put forward the theory innovation of the new concept of cancer metastasis therapy, it was discovered and put forward the third field of human anti-cancer metastasis therapy

-------The circulatory system has a large number of immune surveillance cells, annihilating the transit of cancer cells in the "main battlefield" is in the blood circulation or there are a large number of immune surveillance cells so that it is very important to destroy the cancer cells in the circulation.

⑫ **" The research overview of XZ-C immunocompromised anti-cancer traditional Chinese medications"**

——Using the method of in vitro culture of cancer cells to conduct screening experiments on the inhibition rate of Chinese herbal medicine

——An animal model is made to study the anti-tumor rate of Chinese herbal medicine in cancer-bearing animals

Or

-----In vitro culture of cancer cells, the screening experimental study of the cancer inhibition rate of Chinese herbal medication on of

-----The experimental study on the effect of Chinese herbal medication on the tumor inhibition rate of in tumor-bearing animals

(13) " **the experimental study and clinical efficacy observation of XZ-C immunomodulatory anti-cancer traditional Chinese medication treatment of malignant tumors**"

-------Animal Experiment research and Clinical Application

------ XZ-C immunoregulation anti-cancer traditional Chinese medication is the result of the modernization of traditional Chinese medication

(14) " **the case lists and some typical cases of XZ-C immunoregulation anti-cancer traditional Chinese medication treatment**"

(15) "**cancer treatment reform and innovation research**"

------Adhere to the road of scientific research and innovation of anti - cancer metastasis with Chinese characteristics

-------1 to 8 of the research on cancer treatment reform and innovation

(16) "**walking out of the new way of conquering cancer**"

------ it has formed the theoretical system of XZ-C immune regulation and control and is experiencing clinical application, observation and verification

------ it has had the exclusive research and development products: XZ-C immunoregulation anti-cancer traditional Chinese medication series, has a large number of clinical validation cases

------- 20 years it has walked out of a new way to overcome cancer

6. The next step in cancer research work

(1) our research journey of the ideological understanding and scientific thinking

The journey of ideological awareness and scientific thinking during 28 years of cancer research work research can be divided *into four stages*. Its brief introduction **is that:**

The first stage of 1985 - 1999

- Identify the problem from the follow-up results → ask questions → research questions; **to target the study or to target "in the study of cancer prevention and treatment of postoperative recurrence and metastasis method is the key to improve the long-term efficacy."**

- From the review and the analysis and the reflection, it was found that the current cancer traditional therapies exist the questions, which need to be further studied and improved;

- Recognize the current problems with traditional cancer therapies, and it should change their minds and change the observation;

- the summary of information and the collation and the collection were published the first monograph "new understanding of cancer treatment and new model" in January 2001 Hubei Science and Technology Publishing House.

② the second stage after 2001 -

- Targeting the target of the study and the "target" of cancer therapy is targeted for anti-metastasis and pointing out that the key to cancer treatment is anti-metastasis;

- Conducted a series of new methods of anti - cancer metastasis, recurrence, clinical research and clinical basis and clinical validation, and then ascended into theoretical innovation so that it was propoed the new thinking and new method of ant-cancer metastasis;

- Summary of information, collation, collection, published the second monograph "new concepts and new methods of cancer metastasis therapy" in January 2006 published by the People's Medical Publishing House, Xinhua Bookstore, in April

2007 received the "three one hundred" original book award and certificate issued by the People's Republic of China Press and Publication General.

③ the third stage after 2006 -

- **The research aim and main point are the study of the prevention and treatment during the whole process of cancer occurrence and development;**

- Closely combined with clinical practice, reform and innovation, research and development for the problems and malpractices of current clinical traditional therapies;

- Recognize the strategy of cancer prevention and treatment must move forward, the way out of cancer treatment is in the "three early", anti-cancer out of the way is in the prevention;

- I have been working in oncology for 60 years. The patients are getting more and more. The incidence of cancer is also rising; the death rate is keeping high and no decreasing ; I am deeply aware of that cancer must not only pay attention to treatment, but also pay more attention to prevention. Or I have been engaging in tumor surgery for 60 years, more and more patients, the incidence of cancer is also rising, mortality remains high, so I deeply appreciate that cancer should not only pay attention to treatment, but also pay attention to prevention, in order to stop at the source or it can be blocked at the source; a series of research was carried out ; the information was summarized and organized, collected and published into the third monograph "new concept and new method of cancer treatment" in October 2011 published by the People's Medical Publishing House, Xinhua Bookstore. Followed by American physician Dr. Bin Wu translated into English. The English version of this book was published in USA on March 26, 2013, with international distribution.

④ the fourth stage after 2011 -

Now it is the fourth stage of our research work and is being carried out and developed. _The research work is step by step and the study of the target or "target" is located in reducing the incidence of cancer and improving the cure rate and prolonging the survival time._

We have been working on cancer research for 28 years:

The first three stages of experimental research and clinical research work was mainly in the treatment of new drugs, new methods of diagnosis, new technologies, new concepts and new methods of treatment. The experimental research is mainly to establish a variety of cancer-bearing animal models, to explore the mechanism and law of cancer onset, invasion, recurrence and metastasis, in order to find effective measures to regulate metastasis and recurrence and experimental study on experimental screening of anticancer Chinese herbal medicines for cancer-bearing animals.

But until today the second 10 years of the 21ˢᵗ century, cancer is still rampant, the incidence continues to rise with the high mortality rate. I have been engaged in clinical cancer surgery for 60 years. The more patients are treated and the more patients show up; the incidence of cancer continues to rise so that I deeply appreciate that *in order to stop at the source, it not only pays attention to treatment, but also pays attention to prevention.*

Therefore, I am deeply aware of that the research work of cancer not only focused on the treatment, researching the new drugs and the new methods and the new technologies, but also must focus on how to reduce the incidence of cancer and how to prevent the incidence of cancer from continuing to rise in the momentum?

The current tumor hospital or oncology mode is to go all out to focus on treatment; to aim for patients with the middle or advanced stage diseases, it has poor efficacy and it exhausts human and financial resources, and fails to achieve lower morbidity; the more treatment the more patients. The status quo is: through the road in a century it is a focusing on the treatment and ignoring the defense or the prevention, or there is only treatment but no prevention. Over the years we have just been working and researching cancer treatment. *But in prevention of cancer work it did very little and it almost did not do so that the incidence of cancer continues to rise*.

From the Review and the reflection of the cliché prevention of cancer and the anti-cancer work what have we done in the prevention of cancer research or work since a century? What has the achievement had ?

In the medical school textbooks *teaching content does not attach importance to the knowledge of prevention of cancer*

In hospital mode it does not attach importance to science research program of cancer prevention.

In Journal of Cancer Medical Science there is no paper of paying attention to prevention of cancer.

In short, the prevention of cancer does not attach importance; the prevention of cancer does not pay attention. Cliché prevention is the main, which did not pay attention to and did not implemented.

*How to do? How to reduce the incidence of cancer? How to improve cancer cure **rate? How to reduce cancer mortality?*** How do I extend my life? How to improve the quality of life?

It should launch the total attack of overcoming cancer and both the prevention and the treatment are at the equal attention.

The goal of conquering cancer should be: reduce morbidity, improve the cure rate, reduce mortality, prolong survival, improve quality of life, and reduce complications.

The current global hospitals and the hospitals in China are going all out to engage in treatment and pay attention to the treatment of cancer and ignore the prevention or the defense, or only treatment without the prevention.

XZ-C thinks of that this hospital model or cancer treatment mode can not overcome the cancer, can not reduce the incidence. The global hospitals and our hospital must change the overall strategy of cancer treatment from focusing on cancer treatment into focusing on both the prevention and the treatment.

Therefore, we propose the design and the plans of conquering cancer and launching the total attack to cancer . XZ-C proposed that to launch a total attack, that is,the prevention of cancer **and cancer control and cancer treatment of these three-phase work were developed comprehensively and carried out simultaneously.**

(2)

It was put forward to the "the need and the feasibility of the report to conquer cancer and to launch the general attack on cancer"

It was put forward to " XZ-C research plan to conquer cancer and to launch the total attack of cancer"

The research focus of our 28 years of cancer research in the fourth phase:

After 2011 -

Cancer research work gets deeply step by step

The study objectives and the focuses of the overall strategics of cancer treatment can be changed from focusing on treatment into the prevention and treatment of cancer at the equal attention we proposed to launch the general attack on cancer, that is, the work during three stages of cancer prevention, cancer control, cancer treatment during the whole process of the occurrence and the development of cancer should be developed comprehensive in full swing, simultaneously. That is:

Prevention of cancer - before the formation of cancer

Cancer control - malignant transformation of precancerous lesions

Cancer treatment - has formed a foci or metastases

The general offensive target: to reduce the incidence of cancer, and to reduce cancer mortality, to improve the cure rate, to prolong survival and to improve quality of life and to reduce complications.

The need to launch the general attack of cancer

Why should I make a general attack? Look at the present situation:

1. *the incidence of cancer is the status quo of the more treated the more patients, the new cancer patients of our daily average are 8550 cases, 6 people per minute are diagnosed with cancer in the country*

2. *the status of cancer death is high, has been the first cause of death in urban and rural areas in China, the average daily 7,500 people died of cancer*

3. *the status of treatment, despite the application of the traditional three treatment for nearly a hundred years, tens of thousands of cancer patients bear radiotherapy and chemotherapy, but how are the results? So far the cancer is still the first cause of death.*

4. *the status quo of the current tumor hospital or oncology department of hospital model: pay attention to the treatment and ignore the defense, or only have the treatment. the more treatment the more patients.*

The feasibility of launching attack and capturing cancer

Now is there scientific basis of proposing to launch the total attack of conquering cancer? Is there a medical foundation? Is it possible to win the favorable conditions? Although nearly a century, the traditional therapy failed to conquer cancer, the radiotherapy and the chemotherapy of the traditional therapy can not overcome cancer because it can only alleviate, and can not be cured. But it also made a lot of achievements and experience, and it should further research on the medical basis and expand the results. It is should be feasible and should be timely.

That now it is proposed to launch a total attack has the following scientific basis and medical basis and it is feasible.

Because the United States has finally achieved results in surrendering cancer, because some cancers have found a preventive method, screening can treat some cancers,the prospects for immunomodulatory drugs are gratifying, molecular targeted drugs are eye-catching, advanced cancer has been considered a chronic disease, let the vaccine be used to treat cancer; launching the total offensive and defensive and paying equal attention to the prevention and the treatment will change the status quo; the prevention and control of hepatitis B also become prevention and treatment of liver cancer.

Therefore, the current is the best time and is conducive to propose to conquer cancer and to launch a total attack to cancer.

Xu Ze put forward the "Strategic Thoughts and Suggestions for conquering cancer" in the "New Concepts and New Methods of Cancer Treatment" published in October 2011. In June 2013, Xu Ze proposed "the basic idea and design of conquering cancer and launching the general attack on cancer" in an attempt to reduce the incidence of cancer, reduce mortality, improve the cure rate, prolong survival and the total attack is the prevention of cancer + control cancer + the treatment of the cancer ; the three carriages come hand in hand.

Xu Ze first proposed in the international market in August 2013:

"XZ-C Science Research Plan of conquering cancer and launching the General Attack of Cancer".

This research program was the original innovation and it put forward: the "declared war on cancer" is the time, and it should launch the total attack. To avoid talk and to pay heavy attention to the hard work; no matter how far the path of overcoming cancer is, it should always start to go.

Our dreams are to overcome cancer and to build a well-off society, and everyone is healthy far away from cancer.

- **How to launch the total attack on cancer ?**

XZ-C put forward the idea, strategy, planning diagram of tackling the total attack of cancer and pointed out that the total attack is the work of three stages of the cancer prevention and the cancer control and the cancer treatment which can be developed comprehensively in full swing, simultaneously.

As we all know "how to reduce cancer mortality? How to improve the cure rate? How to extend the survival period?

The way of walking out of cancer treatment is in the "three early" (early detection, early diagnosis, early treatment); the early cancer treatment effect is good and can be cured, especially the precancerous lesions are handled well, and can be cured.

It is now recognized that the <u>occurrence of 90% of cancer</u> has a great relationship with the environmental pollution, although our medical staff go all out in the treatment of cancer; it is still that the more treatment and the more patient and the incidence is indeed rising and it must be blocked at the source. To prevent the occurrence of cancer must try to reduce the incidence rate of cancer.

<u>*The occurrence of cancer is closely related to people's clothing, food, shelter and living habits*</u>. Therefore, I deeply think that it cannot rely on medical staff, and it must rely on the government's major policy; cancer treatment should dependent on medical staff and researchers to study the new drugs and the new diagnostic methods and the new treatment techniques and the new concepts and the new method and new theory of the treatment.

The prevention of cancer and anti-cancer work must rely on the efforts of the government-led and leadership and the experts and the scholars and the masses are involved and the thousands of households participates in order to do.

There are three problems with the current medical profession:

- *First, the more treatment the more patients, the incidence is on the rise, which 90% is related to the environment. We have 28 years of cancer research work (1985 -----)*

*After the review and reflect of experimental research and clinical work, it is deeply appreciated that it is not only paid attention to treatment, but also paid attention to prevention in order to stop at the source, and it must be the prevention and the treatment of cancer at the equal attention. A century ago, the medical pioneers have put forward "prevention of cancer, anti-cancer", but since a century people did not pay attention to the research and measures of cancer prevention. **In 1971 only President Nixon put forward the "anti-cancer slogan" to declare war on cancer.***

- *Second, the current diagnostic methods are behind; B ultrasound, CT, BMI are currently the most advanced diagnostic methods, but once diagnosed, it mostly was in the middle stage and late stage and the effect is very poor. It must seek to the study and to seek the new methods and the new reagents and the new technology of early diagnosis; if it can be diagnosed in the early and precancerous lesions, then early cancer can be cured.*

- *Third, currently some of the patients have the phenomenon of over-diagnosis and over-treatment which the patient has been damaged as so to prompt to reduce immune function of the patients, resulting in disease progression, such as too much CT numbers and too much chemotherapy, it must be paid attention to and be attached the importance to.*

After we experience 28 years of the basis of cancer and clinical research of cancer, it deeply appreciates: to achieve the purpose of cancer prevention and control:

a. It must start the total attack. That is, three stages of work: the cancer prevention and the cancer control and the cancer treatment work together and simultaneously, troika, go hand in hand in order to achieve lower morbidity, improve the cure rate, reduce mortality and prolong survival. If only treatment without prevention or defense, it will never be able to overcome cancer because it cannot reduce the incidence and the more treatment the more patients.

b. **It must be that the government leads and that the experts and the scholars put the efforts and that the masses participate in the mobilization of all and thousands of households participate in order to do. At present, China is building two types of society: the ecological civilization, the energy saving and emission reduction, the pollution prevention and the correction of the pollution prevention; building a well-off society and building an innovation-oriented country are the government-led and the mass participation and the mobilization of the whole people and the thousands of households involved** in the work . It has vigorous development and carrying out and it is a good time, if missed, it will no longer come, if it can conduct the "ride research", it will be able to improve the awareness of anti-cancer in all people to reach the results of preventing cancer and controlling cancer. It gets the effect of decreasing the cancer occurrence rate in our country and our province and the city.

As a result, Prof. Xu Ze presented the following feasibility report and proposal in August 2015.

(1) It was put forward for the first time in the international community:

"the necessity and feasibility report of overcoming cancer and launching the total attack on cancer"

The overall strategic reform of cancer treatment in China should shift the focus of treatment into prevention and treatment at the equal attention

(2) for the first time in the international community **it is put forward :**

"To build prevention and treatment hospital during whole process of cancer occurrence and development

(Global demonstration of cancer prevention and treatment hospital)

"to build the imagination and feasibility report of the prevention and treatment hospital during the anti-cancer whole process"

- Describe the necessity and feasibility of establishing a complete prevention and cure hospital

(3) for the first time in the international community it was put forward :

"To build the imagine of the total attack of conquering cancer and the basic design and feasibility report of the science city"

--is equivalent to design the whole framework with a chinese characteristic design of conquering cancer

(4) for the first time in the international community it was put forward :

"In building a moderately society at the same time, the proposed" ride research "-----to conduct the medical science research of the prevention and the control cancer and the necessity and feasibility report of cancer prevention and treatment"

-- Adhere to the new path of anti - cancer, cancer prevention with the Chinese characteristics of well-off society

These four research projects are the first proposal in the international and is the international initiative and the international leader which opened up a new field of anti-cancer research.

To open up a new field of research will open up a new era of anti-cancer research and will play an epoch-making significance in the course of human anti-cancer research, from the emphasis on the cancer treatment and ignoring the defense into both the prevention and treatment at the same attention in an attempt to reduce cancer incidence rate and to improve the cancer cure rateat the same time.

To open up a new field of research, it is possible to conquer cancer, and even overcome cancer because for a century, in cancer treatment people are based on the treatment, and treatment is based on killing cancer cells. But the chemotherapy is a first-class kinetics and cannot kill cancer cells and can only kill a certain number of cancer cells, there will still have the cancer cells continuing to produce, therefore, its efficacy is set to "ease", and the relief time is only 4 weeks or more. It will still recur and metastasis so chemotherapy cannot cure cancer, although it was used more than half a century, cancer is still the first cause of death of urban and rural residents.

__To propose to conquer cancer and to launch a total attack needs courage and wisdom and strength and scientific basis.__

- Cancer is the enemy of all classes or types. The complexity of cancer is beyond the imagination of human beings, which is the most fiery positions in the field of biomedical and gathers the world's largest and elaborate research team and the scientific research elite.

- Human beings should not sit still, physicians should not do nothing, I think we should put forward the general idea and basic design of attacking cancer and launching the total attack, avoid empty talking, hard work, building a good laboratory, strengthening the experimental research and the basic research and clinical research.

- We have two tasks on the shoulder of the physician: one is to treat the patient, one is the development of medication; we should overcome the cancer in this strategic high-tech field to achieve leapfrog development and to take our characteristics of the technology innovation road of the anti-cancer, anti-transfer and to innovate the achievement and rusults.

- Our doctor has two tasks on the shoulder, one is to treat the patient, the other is to develop medicine; we should achieve leapfrog development in the strategic high-tech field of cancer; take the road of anti-cancer and anti-transfer technology innovation with Chinese characteristics and innovation results.

What should I do next?

This is in need for the government leadership and the government-led and the experts and scholars efforts and the masses involved.

The next step is to work hard and to implement the XZ-C research program; from scratch and from the small to the large, the professional group go hand in hand to carry out, to avoid empty talk, and to do the hard work and to follow the concept of the scientific development with having a plan and having a focus on hard work

The general imagination and design of conquering cancer of how the next step of the work to carry out and achieve the above:

I tentatively envisaged:

How to implement or carry out this new concept and innovation of the prevention and treatment of cancer? A new type of cancer prevention and treatment hospital should be established; the preventing and treating hospitals according to the strategic thinking of preventing and treating cancer occurrence and development during the whole process should be set up. First it creates the model and the demonstration of the Global Prevention and Treatment Hospital.

To overcome cancer must cultivate multidisciplinary senior personnel. From a clinical point of view the following disciplines are related to the research of cancer research:

The immunology and cancer related group;

<u>The virus and cancer related group;</u>

<u>The endocrine and cancer related group;</u>

<u>Fungi and cancer related group;</u>

<u>Chronic inflammation and cancer related group;</u>

<u>Molecular biology and cancer related group;</u>

<u>Gene and cancer related group;</u>

<u>Environment and cancer related group;</u>

<u>Chinese medication and cancer related group.</u>

It is necessary to train senior professionals and intermediate professionals with prevention and control and treatment. Education must cultivate talents for conquering cancer and launching the general attack of cancer and applying what they have learned. It must cultivate the above multidisciplinary senior talents. Talents must have this professional theoretical knowledge and expertise. Talent must be truly practical; talents must have both ability and moral integrity; the talent must be real learning, and <u>the medicine is benevolence and the ethics is the first.</u>

It is recommended to create a trial of the Science City for conquering cancer;

It is recommended to set up a research group of several related groups to overcome cancer;

It is recommended to create a global demonstration or model of the prevention and treatment hospital first;

It is suggested that it must pay attention to the construction of the laboratory. With a good laboratory, it can produce the scientific research results with the original innovation or independent innovation and will help to overcome cancer.

Here, we put forward: "a number of suggestions of the personnel training of the scientific and technological innovation and the laboratory construction, the conversion of the results for the construction of innovative countries". With innovative talent and with a good laboratory the scientific research work in cancer prevention and cancer control and cancer treatment will certainly

achieve fruitful results, and strive to achieve the new results of the prevention and treatment of cancer in China's medical care and strive to achieve a major breakthrough in originality of overcoming cancer in the key areas of the scientific research.

With the continuous improvement of people's living standards, a variety of chemical, physical, biological environment, a large number of carcinogens, a variety of carcinogenic substances come into our body or a variety of carcinogens affect our body so the environment and cancer research, the environmental protection Cancer research will open up the new research areas and the new research industries.

(1) the treatment of malignant tumors appeared twice leap since the last two centuries

Looking back over the past 100 years, the human was suffering from cancer, and so far the formation of cancer is still the lack of the most essential understanding, that is, the normal cell proliferation is subject to what factors control, how they lost control of proliferation and become malignant cells.

In the last two centuries the treatment of malignant tumors has experienced two leaps or there have been two leaps in the treatment of malignant tumors:

The first was that in 1890 Halstad proposed the concept of tumor radicalization; the second time is that in the 1970s Fish integrated chemotherapy into radical surgery (adjuvant chemotherapy or neoadjuvant chemotherapy).

Since then, malignant tumor treatment has been faltering

Fish is a systemic intravenous route that has not been able to reduce mortality and prevent recurrence and metastasis for half a century. Mortality remains the highest.

(2) In 1971, President Nixon issued the "Anti-Cancer Declaration" and proposed anti-cancer slogans in the UN speech.

In 1971, the US Congress passed a "National Cancer Regulations" and President Nixon issued the "Anti-Cancer Declaration." Then it invested considerable human and financial resources to overcome cancer in one fell swoop.

In December 1971, President Richard Nixon presented the anti-cancer slogan in the United Nations.

42 years have passed, and now Nixon has also been ancient, in cancer research has also made many significant progress, such as the discovery of tumor suppressor genes, the advent of monoclonal antibodies, the application of CT and magnetic resonance imaging, the improvement of the ultrasound and endoscopy and the innovation of the various treatment methods .

However, today in the second 10 years of the 21st century the mortality rate of the lung cancer, colon cancer and others of the largest threatening for the human is basically the same as 50 years ago. Cancer deaths are still the first cause of death of urban and rural residents in China.

So the experts in medicine, **biology and related disciplines began to reflect.** *The most scientists believe that the prevention and treatment of the tumor just can get the most effects from the most basic issues, that is, from the nature of cancer cells, pathogenesis, cancer cell metabolic characteristics and signal transduction etc to understand the cancer "Lushan true face", only like this way in order to have the cancer prevention and treatment.*

It should carry out the interdisciplinary research and to promote the basic research and the clinical research cooperation, attention to clinical research.

It must be carried out the clinical basic research and if there is no breakthrough in basic research, the clinical efficacy is difficult to improve.

My third book, "New Concepts and New Methods of Cancer Therapy," have the new concept and innovative content that combines the experimental research and the new concept of clinically proven cancer therapies. It should be implemented in the majority of cancer patients get benefit.

XZ-C proposed the Research Plan of Conquering cancer and Launching the total attack

The overall strategic reform and development of cancer treatment

How to overcome the cancer? I see:

To avoid empty talking, to focus on hard work, no matter how far the path of overcoming cancer it is, it should always start to go.

(one)

- It is time to declare war on cancer, and should start the total attack.

The goal of capturing cancer is to reduce morbidity, reduce mortality, improve cure rate, prolong survival, improve quality of life and reduce complications.

- **To avoid empty talk, to focus on heavy work, no matter how far away the road of capturing cancer it is, it shuld start to go, Wanli Long March always go, thousands of miles began with a single step.**

- What should I do next? Now it was proposed to overcome cancer and to launch a total attack. **It hopes to get leadership support at all levels. I know that to achieve the purpose of cancer prevention, control cancer, cancer treatment must be government leadership, government-led, experts, scholars efforts, the masses to participate in the mobilization of all, thousands of households to participate in order to do.**

- Recognize that more than 90% of the cancer is caused by or closely related to environmental factors. **Building a well-off society and anti-cancer, cancer control has a great relevance, therefore, we propose to prevent the cancer and to launch a total attack, adhere to the Chinese characteristics of anti-cancer, cancer prevention path.**

- At present, China's country is implementing the spirit of the 18th Party Congress and comprehensively building a well-off society to ensure the goal of achieving a well-off society in 2020. **Our dreams, to overcome cancer, to build a well-off society, everyone is healthy and away from cancer.**

(two)

- Why did I propose to launch a total attack? Why is it urgent? Look at the current situation: (according to the National Cancer Registration Center released the "2012 China Cancer Registration Annual Report"

- the status quo of the incidence of cancer is that the more treatment the more patients, our average daily new cancer patients is for the 8550 cases, 6 persons per minute are confirmed as cancer in the national.

- **the status of cancer mortality** is high, has been the first cause of death in urban and rural areas, 7,500 people died of cancer in the average daily.

- **the status of treatment**, despite the application of the traditional three treatment for nearly a hundred years, tens of thousands of cancer patients bear the chemotherapy and chemotherapy, but what are the results? So far the cancer is still the first cause of death.

- **the current situation of the hospital mode** is to pay attention to treatment with the light defense or prevention, or only treatment without prevention, the more treatment the more patients.

The status quo is: **a century through the road is a heavy treatment and light defense, or only treatment . Anti-cancer is the career of mankind**, but over the years we have just studied on cancer treatment, but do little work on cancer prevention, almost did not do.

- Therefore, XZ-C suggests that the general idea and overall design of the cancer should be launched, as well as the overall planning, route, and blueprint.

On the treatment of cancer it must have a whole strategic reform from light defense or prevention into for both of the prevention and treatment at the same attention.

It should update their minds, update their knowledge, move forward in reform, innovate in reform, and develop in reform.

(three)

- Cancer is the enemy of all mankind and should arouse the common struggle of mankind around the world. The complexity of cancer is beyond human imagination, which is the hottest position in biomedicine, gathering the world's largest, elite research team and research elite.

- To tackle cancer as the main direction of the study, experimental and clinical anti-cancer research should be a key area of scientific research, should achieve an original breakthrough.

- There are 2.7 million cases of cancer deaths each year, with an average of 7,500 deaths per day in cancer. Such amazing data should be included as scientific research in key areas of scientific and technological innovation.

- Human beings should not sit still, physicians should not do nothing, I think we should propose to the general idea and basic design of capturing cancer, "declared war on cancer" and launch a total attack. **To avoid the empty talk, to pay attention to heavy hard work, building a good laboratory, to strengthen experimental research, basic research and clinical research.**

- **We have two tasks on the shoulder of the physician, one is to treat the patient, one is the development of medicine, we should overcome the cancer in this strategic high-tech field to achieve leapfrog development,** take our characteristics of anti-cancer, anti-transfer technology innovation Road, innovation, and strive to enter the forefront of the world.

- Because cancer patients are getting more and more, the morbidity is on the rise, the mortality rate is high, recognizing that cancer should not only pay attention to treatment, but also pay attention to prevention, in order to stop at the source, is the research goal and focus on the occurrence of cancer, Development of the whole process of prevention and control of the study.

Xu ZE in October 2011 published in Beijing, "new concepts and new methods of cancer treatment," Chapter 38 of the proposed "to overcome the strategic thinking of cancer and suggestions." The book was later published by the American medical scientist Dr. Bin Wu and other English, the English version published in March 26, 2013 in Washington, the international distribution.

In June 2013 Xu Ze also put forward the " the general idea and design to conquer cancer and launch the total attacka " in an attempt to reduce the incidence of cancer, reduce mortality, improve the cure rate, prolong survival.

"XZ-C proposed the research project of conquering the cancer and launching a total attack"

The overall strategic reform and development of cancer treatment

Prof. Xu ZE, Honorary President of Wuhan Anti-Cancer Research Association, presented the following feasibility report and proposal in July 2015.

(1) It was put forward for the first time in the international community:

"The necessity and feasibility report of overcoming cancer and launching the total attack on cancer"

-------The overall strategic reform of cancer treatment is to shift the focus of treatment into prevention and treatment at the equal attention

(2) for the first time in the international community it is put forward :

"To build prevention and treatment hospital during whole process of cancer occurrence and development"

(Global demonstration of cancer prevention and treatment hospital)

"To build the imagination and feasibility report of the prevention and treatment hospital during the anti-cancer whole process"

----- *Describe the necessity and feasibility of establishing a complete prevention and cure hospital*

(3) *for the first time in the international community it was put forward :*

"To build the imagine of conquering cancer and launch the total attack and the basic design and feasibility report of the science city"

- is equivalent to design the whole framework with a chinese characteristic design of conquering cancer

(4) *for the first time in the international community it was put forward :*

"In building a moderately society at the same time, the proposed" *ride research* **"-----conduct the medical science research of the prevention and the control cancer and the necessity and feasibility report of cancer prevention and treatment"**

- Adhere to the new path of anti - cancer, cancer prevention with the Chinese characteristics of well-off society

These four research projects are the first proposal in the international and are the international initiative and the international leader which opened up a new field of anti-cancer research.

To shift from paying attention to cancer treatment and ignoring prevention into paying attention to both the treatment and prevention, try to decrease the cancer incidence rate, to increase the cancer cure rate.

To open up a new field of research is possible to conquer cancer, and even overcome cancer.

The necessity and the feasibility for conquering cancer and launching the general attack of cancer

<u>The overall strategic reform of china's cancer treatment shifts from focusing on treatment to focusing on both cancer prevention and treatment at the equal attention</u>

Cancer is a common enemy of all mankind, should mobilize the world's scientists, leaders, the masses involved in research to overcome cancer, should call the global mobilization to capture cancer, the current is the time, it is urgent.

<u>The goal of conquering cancer</u> is to reduce morbidity, reduce mortality, improve cure rate, prolong survival, improve quality of life and reduce complications.

The current treatment of cancer hospital or cancer cancer mainly concentrated in the late stage, the treatment effect is poor.

The walk-out of Cancer treatment is in **the "three early", early detection, early diagnosis, early treatment.** Early treatment of patients has good results and improves the treatment effect so that it is necessary to reduce the mortality rate of cancer, improve the cure rate.

If we can do cancer treatment very well in the precancerous lesions or early stage, then the patients who progress to the invasion and metastasis and the late stages will be reduced, which is to reduce the incidence of cancer.

If you ignore the precancerous lesions, early patients, it is impossible to reduce the incidence of cancer. The key to cancer treatment is in the "three early", and how to deal with precancerous lesions, it is a critical stage of cancer prevention and treatment.

I have been engaged in clinical cancer surgery for 60 years, the more treatment and the more patients, the incidence of cancer is also rising, so I deeply appreciate that cancer should not only pay attention to treatment, but also pay attention to prevention, in order to stop at the source.

Cancer is not only a serious threat to human health, but also an important factor in the rapid rise in medical costs. China's annual cancer treatment with the direct cost of nearly 100 billion yuan, so that patients and the whole society to bear a huge financial burden.

Although countries spend a lot of money on the treatment of cancer patients, but the past 20 years, some of the common 5-year survival of cancer has not improved significantly. For example, in the United States from 1974 to 1990, the 5-year survival rate of esophageal cancer rose from only 7% to 9%, gastric cancer from 16% to 19%, liver cancer from 3% to 6%, lung cancer from 12% to 15% Pancreatic cancer is basically no change is still 3%.

How to do? The way out of conquering cancer is prevention.

For malignant tumors, prevention is better than cure. Through the adjustment of public health resources and strategies, strategic shift, the focus shifted from treatment to prevention, both cancer prevention and treatment at the equal attention, to carry out active and effective early warning, early diagnosis and intervention study to reduce the incidence of cancer and improve the cure rate, has become a global cancer research The consensus of the workers.

How to fight cancer? How to overcome cancer?

XZ-C proposed the overall design and overall attack design, as well as the overall attack planning, route, blueprint of attacking the cancer and launch the attack.

What is so-called total attack? That is the three carriages such as the prevention of cancer and cancer control and cancer treatment which keep pace together and run together and put both the cancer prevention and treatment at the same level.

The overall strategic reform of focusing on cancer treatment and light prevention shifts into the emphasis on the cancer prevention and treatment at the same level and attention and both the prevention and anti-cancer are put at the same time and at the same level, which should be updated thinking and updated awareness;

it is to progress in the reform and to be the innovation in the reform and to be the development in the reform.

1. XZ-C proposed to the general idea and design of conquering cancer

----- XZ-C (XU ZE - China)

(1) What is the total attack on conquering cancer?

The total attack is to develop the comprehensive work of the three stages such as the prevention cancer and control cancer and treatment of cancer during the whole process of the occurrence and development of cancer in full swing and simultaneously.

That is:

The prevention of cancer - before the formation of cancer

The controlling cancer - malignant transformation of precancerous lesions

The treatment of cancer - has formed a foci or metastases

The main goal:

To reduce the incidence of cancer, to reduce cancer death, to improve the cure rate, to prolong survival, to improve quality of life, to reduce complications.

Xu Ze (XU ZE) Professor proposed the general offensive ideas, strategies, planning of overcoming cancer and launch a total attach as follows:

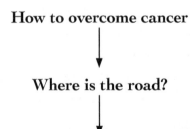

How to overcome cancer

↓

Where is the road?

↓

Our ideas, strategies, planning should be divided into three parts (or three stages)

↓

Aiming for the whole process of the occurrence and the development of cancer to do prevention and treatment

↓

Before the formation of cancer - for the prevention part - anti-mutation

↓

There may be malignant tendencies of precancerous lesions - for the intervention part

↓

The treatment of primary cancer that has foci is treated with anti-metastatic treatment

↓

Prevention of susceptible stage   precancerous stage   cancer and metastasis

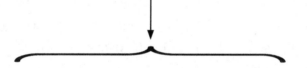

Early   non-metastasis   has been transferred

↑   ↑   ↑

Prevention of cancer   control cancer   treatment of cancer

(2) Why did I put forward to the total attack?

The current tumor hospital or oncology departments all pay attention to heavy treatment and light prevention or only treatment without prevention.

I entered the Zhongnan Tongji Medical College in 1951, so far 65 years, experienced and witnessed the whole process of the prevention and treatment of cancer in China for a century. Review of the 20th century, China and the global hospitals, although it also mentioned to prevent cancer and anti-cancer work, but in fact the focus has been formed in the primary cancer treatment and anti-metastatic treatment of cancer, which are in the invasion period, the middle and the late stages ; the treatment effect is poor.

So far to the second decade of the 21ˢᵗ century, the world's hospitals, China's provincial cancer hospital, the hospital affiliated hospital oncology, the three level hospitals are cancer treatment hospital, tumor hospital are clinical treatment. The modes of building the hospitals are all for the treatment of hospitals, oncology academic journals are also clinically diagnosis or clinically based, although there are several for the cancer prevention magazine, but very few anti-cancer work articles. In short, the 20ᵗʰ century, the tumor hospital and the university affiliated hospital of the tumor are heavy treatment, or only treatment without prevention .

Review, reflection, cliché anti-cancer, anti-cancer work, for a century what have we done in the prevention-cancer research or work? What achievement did you have?

The status quo is: a century through the road is to pay attention to treatment and light prevention, or only treatment. Prevention of cancer, anti-cancer is the undertaking or cause of mankind, but over the years we do only in the anti-cancer and cancer treatment research work. But in prevention of cancer work was done very little, almost did not do.

Medical school textbooks teaching content does not attach importance to prevention of cancer knowledge.

The hospital mode of building hospital does not attach importance to set up work of prevention of cancer science.

Medical school or hospital research projects do not attach importance to prevention of cancer research projects. Journal of Oncology has not paid attention to prevention of cancer work papers. In short, prevention of cancer does not attach importance; the prevention of cancer was not pay attention to.

Cliché anti-cancer, anti-cancer work, cliché prevention of cancer is as the main point, which was not paid attention to and not implemented.

(3) how to launch the total attack on conquering cancer?

XZ-C (Xu Ze-China) proposed to launch the total attack, that is, three stages of work : prevention of cancer, cancer control, and cancer treatment are carried out comprehensively and implemented simultaneously.

As we all know: how to reduce cancer mortality rate? How to improve the cure rate? How to extend life?

The walking-out of cancer treatment is in the "three early" (early detection, early diagnosis, early treatment); the effect of the early cancer treatment is good, can be cured completely, especially if cancer lesions are handled well, all of them can be cured completely.

How to overcome the cancer I see:

2. The necessity of launching the total attack to conquering cancer

Why should I propose to launch a general attack? Why is it that there is no time to delay? The current status: Please look at the current situation:

(1) The current situation of cancer incidence is that the more patients are treated, the more patients; the current incidence of cancer in China is 3.12 million new cases of cancer every year. On average 8550 new cancer patients were diagnosed every day, and 6 people were diagnosed with cancer every minute in the country.

(2) the status quo of cancer mortality is high, has been the first cause of death in urban and rural areas in China, the annual death of cancer cases, 2.7 million people, an average of 7,500 people died of cancer every day, every 7 dead 1 person died of cancer.

(3) the status of treatment

Although the application of the traditional three treatments has been for nearly a hundred years, tens of thousands of cancer patients used the radiotherapy and chemotherapy, but how are the results? So far the cancer is still the first cause of death, although the patient used the formal, systematic radiotherapy and / or chemotherapy, or radiotherapy and chemotherapy, it still failed to prevent cancer metastasis, recurrence,

(4) the current tumor hospital or oncology mode of the status quo

① go all out to focus on treatment, for the middle stage or the late stage and poor efficacy, exhausted human and financial resources, and failed to achieve lower mortality, improve the cure rate, reduce morbidity.

② only treatment, or heavy treatment with light defense, the more treatment and the more patients.

③ Ignored the "three early", ignoring the precancerous lesions.

④ neglected prevention.

⑤ **people**: while talking about cancer, the skin color changes

Patient, family members: helpless or no hope

Doctors and nurses:

Powerless, medical treatment stay in the three treatments, the effect is wandering and doesn't move forward.

The attitude of people understanding:

A variety of chemical, physical, biological environment carcinogens appears in a large number, a variety of carcinogenic substances into the human body or a variety of carcinogens affect the human body, people seem to be shrouded in the environment of carcinogens in the ocean; while some people talk about cancer, the skin color changes. It seems that all of the vegetation are soldiers, some people are insensitive, goes its own way in the life of their own way. *Cancer is not terrible, terrible is that we do not have this simple knowledge. With this basic knowledge, most of the cancer can be avoided and can be prevented.*

⑥ many large hospitals, university affiliated hospitals have not established a laboratory, cannot carry out basic research or basic clinical research of cancer, because if no basic research breakthrough, the clinical efficacy is difficult to improve. *"Oncology" is still the most backward in the current medical disciplines, why? Because the etiology, pathogenesis, pathophysiology of "oncology" are not yet clear.* The pathogenesis and cancer cell metastasis mechanism are still lack of understanding and the complex biological behavior of cancer cells is still lack of sufficient understanding, and therefore the current treatment program is still quite blind, it must establish a laboratory for basic research and clinical basis the study.

3. *The feasibility of conquering cancer and launching the total attack*

Is there any scientific basis for launching a general attack on cancer? Is there a medical basis? Are there any favorable conditions for winning?

Although traditional treatments have failed to conquer cancer, traditional treatments, and chemotherapy have not been able to overcome cancer for nearly a century, because it can only be alleviated and cannot be cured, but it has also achieved many results and experience, which should be based on this medicine. However, many achievements and experiences have been achieved, and in-depth research should be conducted on this medical basis to expand the results.

(1) *human beings has made great achievements in the surrender of cancer*

Since December 1971, when the then president of the United States Nongsong signed the "National Cancer Act", is considered a human war on cancer officially declared.

Fortunately, 42 years have passed, reviewing its achievements, shows that humans have made great achievements in surrendering cancer: statistics show that the incidence of cancer in the United States since 1996 began to decline significantly, cancer mortality since 1990 Has fallen by 17%, cancer 5-year survival rate increased by 18%, made significant new results, indicating that cancer is likely to be gradually surrendered.

(2) *Now some of the cancer found a prevention method*

①The study is found that ***chronic inflammation*** is the leading cause of cervical cancer, liver cancer, gastric cancer, the main reason for cervical cancer is based on chronic cervicitis; liver cancer is based on chronic hepatitis or cirrhosis; gastric cancer mostly is based on chronic gastritis, or gastric ulcer. Prevention of these parts of the inflammation or eradication of cancer pathogenic factors (such as stomach, colon cancer treatment of Helicobacter pylori) may prevent the occurrence of cancer.

②It is well known ***that lifestyle is one of the key factors in the pathogenesis of cancer, especially tobacco.*** Promoting smoking bans and healthy eating habits can prevent lung cancer and other cancers. The lifestyle that promotes cancer prevention is: Non-smoking, limited alcohol, lose weight.

(3) *screening can prevent or treat part of the cancer*

① **colorectal cancer is the basis of polyp**, remove the polyps can prevent the occurrence of cancer, and colonoscopy screening can reduce the incidence of colorectal cancer and mortality. Where there are intestinal symptoms or blood in the stool it should have colonoscopy.

② **cervical smears can be effectively found in cervical precancerous lesions, through the treatment of precancerous lesions it can prevent cancer.**

③The mammography X-ray can screen for early breast cancer.

Most of the above three cancers can be cured if they are detected early, the vast majority can be cured.

(4) *The prospect of immunomodulatory drugs is gratifying*

Regardless of the complexity of the mechanisms behind cancer, immune suppression is the key to cancer progression. Removing the immunosuppressive factor and restoring the recognition of cancer cells by body or systemic cells can effectively prevent cancer. More and more research evidence shows that by regulating the body's immune system, it is possible to achieve the goal of controlling cancer.Treating tumors by activating the body's anti-tumor immune system is an area that is currently exciting for researchers. The next major breakthrough in cancer is likely to come from this.

In order to explore the etiology, pathogenesis and pathophysiology of cancer, we have carried out a series of animal experimental studies. From the experimental results, we have obtained new findings and new revelation: thymus atrophy and immune function are one of the causes and pathogenesis of cancer so Xu Ze (Xu Ze) professor proposed at the international conference that one of the pathogenesis and etiology may be thymus atrophy, central immune sensory dysfunction, immune dysfunction, immune surveillance capacity decline and immune escape.

As a result of laboratory study it was found that: in the cancer-bearing mice thymus was atrophic atrophy, central immune sensory function damage, decreased immune function, immune surveillance is low, so the treatment principle must be to prevent thymus atrophy, promote thymus Hyperplasia, protection of bone marrow hematopoietic function to improve immune surveillance, for the immune regulation of cancer provides a theoretical basis and experimental basis.

Based on the above research on the cause and pathogenesis of cancer, the new idea and new method of XZ-C immunoregulation therapy are put forward. After 30 years of cancer specialist outpatient clinic more than 12,000 cases of advanced cancer patients with clinical validation, it was confirmed that the principle of treatment of promotion of Thymus proliferation and increase of immune function is reasonable, the effect is satisfactory. Application of immune regulation and control of traditional

Chinese medicine has achieved good results, improved the quality of life, significantly extended the survival period.

XZ-C (XU ZE-China) immunomodulation method was first proposed by Professor Xu Ze in his book "New Concepts and New Methods of Cancer Metastasis Treatment" in 2006. He believes that under normal circumstances, there is a dynamic balance between cancer and body defense. The occurrence of cancer is caused by an imbalance in dynamic balance. If the state has been adjusted to a normal level, it can control the growth of cancer and cause cancer to subside.

It is well known *that the occurrence, progression and prognosis of cancer is determined by a combination of two factors, that is, the biological characteristics of cancer cells and the host organism itself*, the ability to control cancer cells, such as it is the balance between the two, the cancer can be controlled, if both Imbalance, cancer will develop.

Under normal circumstances, the host of the body itself has a certain ability to control cancer cells, but in the presence of cancer, these control defensive ability to varying degrees of inhibition and damage, resulting in cancer cells lost immune surveillance, the occurrence of cancer immune escape, Making cancer cells further development, metastasis.

Through the above four years to explore the recurrence and metastasis mechanism of the basic experimental study, and after 3 years from the natural medicine herbal experiments in vivo through the tumor in vivo tumor inhibition test, from the herbal medicine to screen out a number of good tumor inhibition rate of traditional Chinese medications. They were composed of XZ-C$_{1-10}$ anti-cancer immune regulation and control of traditional Chinese medications .

(5) *The molecular targeted drug therapy is eye-catching*

In 1960, Philadelphia researchers found that there was a chromosomal abnormality in patients with chronic myeloid leukemia (CML). Years later, the researchers found that this was the results of a chromosome 9 and 22 chromosome long-arm translocation. **Since this chromosomal abnormality was first found at the expense (Philadelphia), it was named the Philadelphia (ph) chromosome**. The chromosome has also become a target for CML targeted therapy for 40 years. In 2001 the first confirmed to be against Philadelphia chromosome molecular defects - imatinib.

Followed by the human epidermal growth factor receptor 2 (HER2) as the target targeting drug Quartin monoclonal antibody, the treatment of HER2-positive breast cancer, VEGF as the target of paclitaxel and EGFR as the target Cetuximab treatment of colorectal cancer. The targets of EGFR are as gefitinib and erlotinib for non - small cell lung cancer treatment.

Molecular targeted drugs are cell stabilizers, most patients can not achieve CR, PR, but the condition is stable and improve the quality of life. Besides the foritidine, erlotinib, imatinib, the need to use in combination with chemotherapy drugs.

Molecular targeting drugs represent a new class of anti-cancer drugs, and imatinib (Gleevec) is a typical example that can control cancer by inhibiting abnormal molecules that cause cancer, without damaging other normal nuclei. There have been a growing number of molecular targeted drugs for the treatment of cancer, such as B cell lymphoma of rituximab (Rituximab) treatment of breast cancer trastuzumab (Trastuzumab) and the treatment of lung cancer Nepal (Gifitinib) erlotinib (Erlotinib) and so on. Targeted therapy brings anti-tumor hope.

(6) *Advanced cancer has been considered chronic disease*

Like high bloodness, coronary heart disease, advanced cancer has a variety of drug options, there are many kinds of molecular targeted drugs as a candidate, as well as biological therapy, immunotherapy, immunomodulation therapy, integrated traditional Chinese and Western medicine treatment, through the above joint treatment, it can survive with the tumor, some patients with advanced cancer can also survive for many years.

(7) *to make the application of vaccine treatment of cancer as possible, human papillomavirus (HPV) can cause cervical cancer and HPV vaccine was found*

In 1983, Professor Hausen found a new HPVDNA in the cervical cancer biopsy to find the new HPV16 virus. In 1984, HPV16 and HPV18 were cloned from cervical cancer patients, and later proved worldwide About 70% of cervical cancer patients are carrying both viruses.

In 1991, a large epidemiology confirmed that HPV was a causative agent for cervical cancer. HPV vaccine research started, and into clinical research.

In June 2006, preventive vaccines for cervical cancer were approved by the US Food and Drug Administration (FDA).

HPV vaccine is divided into two kinds of preventive vaccines and therapeutic vaccines, the current success of the study is a preventive vaccine.

HPV infection caused by cervical cancer can be vaccinated to prevent, which makes people finally realize the dream of having cancer vaccine.

(8) *To launched the total attack and the prevention and treatment of cancer at the same attention which will change the status quo*

Cancer has been beyond the cardiovascular and cerebrovascular diseases and become the primary cause of death of urban and rural people which is mainly due to heavy treatment and the light prevention or defense, and even only treatment ; census is not a wide range of promotion and the proportion of early diagnosis of cancer is low and it did not attach importance to the three early and to the treatment of precancerous lesions. As well as the effectiveness of the ban on smoking and the growing environmental pollution are getting worse. It can be expected, China's cancer prevention and control situation in the future for a long time is still grim. In view of this situation, it should be proposed to attack the cancer and launch a total attack, that is, the prevention of cancer, cancer control, treatment, Troika go hand in hand, prevention and treatment at the same attention will gradually change the status quo.

(9) *hepatitis B prevention and control, that is, is to do the prevention and treatment of primary liver cancer and the primary liver cancer in China occurred on the basis of liver cirrhosis lesions*

Hepatitis B → slow live liver → liver stiffness → portal hypertension → {
Enlarged spleen

Acites

Jaundice

Hepatic encephalopathy
}

To prevent and treat primary liver cancer should be appropriate to prevent hepatitis B.

Hepatitis B (hepatitis B) not only seriously affects the health of patients, but also the family and the community which caused a heavy economic burden, is harmful to the health of the people of the important public health problems. China is a high incidence of hepatitis B in 1992, the national epidemiological survey of hepatitis B showed that the population of chronic hepatitis B virus (HBV) carrying rate of 9.75%, that is, every one of 10 people for hepatitis B.

Prevention of the occurrence of primary liver cancer s necessary to prevent liver cirrhosis caused by hepatitis B. Hepatitis B and cirrhosis of the patients are high-risk groups and should be actively treated to prevent its malignant.

The newborns vaccination of hepatitis B vaccine is an important measure to control hepatitis B, through the implementation of neonatal hepatitis B vaccination, effectively protect the children infected with HBV, hepatitis B prevention and control significantly.

Prevention and control of hepatitis B also prevention and treatment of liver cancer caused by hepatitis B cirrhosis.

4. The current is the best time and is conducive to put forward conquering cancer and launching a total attack.

(1) At present, China is building an innovative country, is the prosperity of scientific and technological innovation, the National Science and Technology Innovation Conference deepened the reform of science and technology system, decided to enter the ranks of innovative countries in 2020, its goal for key areas of scientific research achieves a major breakthrough. Strategic high-tech fields achieve leapfrog development; a number of areas of new achievements went into the forefront of the world; universal scientific quality generally improved, into the ranks of innovative countries.

How to build an innovative country? Innovative countries should not only prosper their own innovation, but also prosperity of the original innovation, not only catch the international advanced level, but also reach the international leading level.

Cancer is the enemy of all mankind, the complexity of cancer beyond human imagination, which is the hottest field of biomedical position, gathered the world's largest elite research team and research elites.

Cancer is not a disease, but a similar feature of a wide range of diseases, although cancer treatment has been more than a century, now it enters the first two decades of the 21st century, but "oncology" is still the most backward of a discipline in the current medical subjects, why? Because the etiology, pathogenesis, pathophysiology of the "oncology" of are not yet clear. Oncology for scientific research, is a virgin land and need to conduct a lot of basic scientific research and clinical basic research.

To overcome the cancer as the main direction of the study and to do the experimental and clinical anti-cancer research should be the key areas of scientific research to achieve the original breakthrough.

According to the National Cancer Registration Center released the "2012 China Cancer Registration Annual Report", the annual number of new cases of cancer is about 312 million cases, an average of 8550 people a day, the country every 6 people diagnosed with cancer.

There are 2.7 million cases of cancer deaths per year, with an average of 7,500 deaths per day. Such amazing data should be included as scientific research in key areas of scientific and technological innovation.

Human beings should not sit still, physicians should not do nothing, I think we should put forward the general idea of conception of cancer and basic design of "declared war on cancer" which is the time and it should launch the total attack.

We have two tasks on the shoulder of the physician, one is to treat the patient, one is the development of medication, we should overcome the cancer in this strategic high-tech field to achieve leapfrog development, take our characteristics of anti-cancer anti-transfer technology innovation path, Innovation, and strive to enter the forefront of the world.

My second book "new concepts and new methods of cancer metastasis therapy", was published in January 2006, Beijing People's Medical Publishing House, Xu Ze with. In April 2007 a "three hundred" original book certificate was issued by the People's Republic of China .

My third book "new concept and new method of cancer treatment" was published in October 2011 Beijing. By People's Medical Publishing House, Xu Ze, Xu Jie. It was Followed by that American medical doctor Dr. Bin Wu translated into English, the English version in March 26, 2013 published in Washington, the international distribution.

(2) the current province and the city are in accelerating the realization of Wuhan city circle "two-oriented society" construction of a new breakthrough and the Wuhan is built as a national center city. In this excellent situation, we should grasp the

national implementation of the strategy to promote the rise of the central region and the Wuhan city circle "two-oriented society" comprehensive reform of the sincere construction of new areas of great opportunity to blaze new trails. I deeply think that: in this excellent situation, great opportunity, it also creates a good opportunity for cancer prevention and cancer control research work,. Therefore, I suggest: you can engage in "ride scientific research", never missed; if missed, the time will no longer come.

What is "riding car scientific research"?

This is what I think, no one mentioned in the literature. The current rise of the central strategy and the construction of "two-oriented society", is a historic great initiative: is the great initiative of the great country and the people ; is the power in the current and the benefits are in the future; it is the greatness of welfare for the health benefits of hundreds of millions of people. I would like to take a "scientific research train" under this great historical wheel to engage in the prevention of cancer, anti-cancer research work done up will receive fruitful results and may even get "two-oriented society" new breakthrough.

I think the current energy-saving emission reduction and pollution prevention and control and "build two-type society" are I-level prevention to prevent cancer prevention. Its purpose and effect can reach the level of prevention of cancer I level. This is a golden opportunity, it must lap this golden opportunity; if missed, it will no longer come. I have been engaged in the experimental study of tumor surgery and clinical practice for half a century. It is deeply to realize that in order to reach the purpose of cancer prevention and control it must be government-led, experts, scholars efforts, the masses to participate in the mobilization of all, thousands of households to participate in order to do. And now the province and the city are the rise of the central strategy of the in-depth implementation of the national central city and the "two-oriented society" construction, it is government-led, the masses to participate in the mobilization of all the thousands of households involved in the work; it must improve the cancer awareness to achieve the effects of the prevention of cancer and cancer control and to receive to the effect of significantly reducing cancer incidence rate, which is the Chinese characteristics of "two types of society" anti-cancer, cancer prevention path.

Therefore, the current is the most time, is conducive for us to attack the cancer and to launch a total attack.

(3) At present, China is implementing the spirit of the 18th National Congress and meeting the well-off society to ensure the goal of building a well-off society in an all-round way in 2020.

The main contents are "the significant progress in resource-saving and environment-friendly society construction and the total discharge of major pollutants is significantly reduced and the stability of the ecosystem is enhanced and the people's environment has improved obviously."

Strengthen the natural ecosystem and environmental protection efforts, adhere to the prevention of the main, comprehensive management, to address the environmental health of the people seriously focus on the focus.

Building a well-off society and people improve their health knowledge and the environmental pollution and other pathogenic factors have the effective intervention will reduce the incidence of cancer-related.

Recognize that more than 90% of the cancer are caused or closely related to the environmental factors. Building a well-off society has a great relevance to the prevention of cancer and cancer control, therefore, we propose to attack the cancer and launch a total attack, to adhere to the Chinese characteristics of anti-cancer and cancer prevention path.

In the building of a moderately prosperous society, rural urbanization work, it is to develop the prevention of cancer and anti-cancer outline and it is put forward and develop the prevention of cancer and anti-cancer measures. It is to develop the cancer prevention and control planning and measures in the new towns, new rural.

Recognize the building of a well-off society should be everyone healthy, away from cancer, anti-cancer out of the way lies in the prevention; in the rural urbanization in China it is to carry out the prevention of cancer, anti-cancer work and to adhere to the path of Chinese characteristics of the prevention of cancer, anti-cancer. It is put forward the necessity of launching the total attack.

Our dreams are to conquer cancer, build a well-off society, everyone healthy, away from cancer.

5. <u>**To avoid empty talking about, to pay attention to heavy hard work, no matter how far away the road to attack cancer it is, it should always start to go**</u>

What should I do next? Now it is proposed to overcome cancer and launch a total attack. Hope to get leadership support at all levels. We must know how to achieve the purpose of cancer prevention and control, we must be government leaders, government-led, experts, scholars efforts, the masses to participate in the mobilization of all nations, thousands of households to participate in order to do so.

(1) regardless of the way to overcome the cancer how far, how long it is, it should always start to go, always go to the long march, thousands of miles begins with a single step. Miles long march, it should start the start, as long as the forward, the grass will always come out of a way, the focus is to avoid empty talking about and to keep the hard work, hard work can be a result and the hard work is to act. The current status quo is to focus on treatment an light defense, or only treatment; To overcome the cancer should be launched a total attack and the prevention of cancer, cancer control, cancer treatment three carriages go hand in hand; go hand in hand - vigorously experiment, vigorously practice, hard work.

How to work? "Conducting scientific research on cancer control and prevention to develop plans and measures for cancer control" (see another article)

(2) the current situation is difficult main point, but it should also start

To promote research and experiment and to call for mobilization of the whole people, to promote the capture of cancer, to launch a total attack, to launch the prevention of cancer, cancer control, cancer treatment, three carriages go hand in hand to launch the total attack. The whole people appeal to improve the prevention of cancer, cancer control knowledge, related to the real interests of each person, in order to achieve awareness of conquering cancer, it must mobilize the whole people, the whole people work, I know that to achieve this goal, we must arouse the people; to overcome the cancer, we must mobilize all the people to mobilize, a mighty force, government leadership, government-led, expert efforts, the masses to participate in order to do.

(3) why is it today to launch a total attack? No time to wait, have to propose to launch a total attack ; and the opportunity cannot be missed and it have to propose to launch the total attack.

The original hope that in the modern oncology, the traditional three treatment can conquer and even overcome cancer; now it appears that is can not rely on chemotherapy to overcome cancer, after 30 years of clinical practice gradually believe that radiotherapy and chemotherapy cannot overcome cancer, because it exists Many problems and drawbacks, it can only alleviate, that is, short-term improvement, can not be cured. It can only be used as adjuvant therapy, cannot cure, can only palliative (may be shortened some).

That is being the case, it should find another way, launch a total attack, take a new road. The whole treatment = surgery + biotherapy + immunoregulation therapy + Chinese and Western combination therapy + targeted therapy. The short-term treatment = radiotherapy +chemotherapy as the supplemented (not long-range, not excessive)

The way-out of Cancer treatment is in the "three early", the way out of anti-cancer is in the prevention.

1/3 of the cancer can be prevented. It should pay attention to the basis of precancerous lesions and clinical diagnosis and treatment technology research. The road of scientific research is to carry out multidisciplinary research, special in-depth basis and clinical disciplines, and it should be woven with the specialist group which is closely related to a number of cancer, special in-depth basis and clinical research.

6. The total and general idea of how to carry out and achieve the above capture of cancer

① Professor Xu Ze proposed the proposal of "the establishment of the National Cancer Working Group,", and "province, city attack cancer work group (station)" first pilot experiment (see another article).

It was Proposed to create "to overcome the Cancer Science City" test (see another article).

The recommendations to conquer cancer is to set up several research group (see another article)

It is First create a global model of the hospital for prevention and treatment (see another article).

"Declaring war on cancer" is the time and should start the total attack. That is, the prevention of cancer, cancer control, cancer treatment three carriages go hand in hand, at the same time to carry out prevention and treatment both. The prevention of cancer and cancer control goal are to reduce the incidence of cancer ; the prevention goal is to reduce mortality, improve the cure rate, prolong survival, live long, good quality of life.

② to capture cancer and to launch a total attack, personnel training is the key (see another article)

It is necessary to cultivate high-level professionals and intermediate professionals with prevention, control and governance. Personnel must have this specialist knowledge and technology. At present, multidisciplinary comprehensive treatment is necessary. Talent must be true to learn, talent must both ability and political integrity. Training personnel must pay attention to the construction of the laboratory; with a good laboratory, it is to have the main innovation or the original innovation of scientific research. With the laboratory, it can have the talent and have the scientific research results.

<u>With the results of scientific and technological innovation, we must promptly transform into clinical medicine to improve the level of medical care, so that patients benefit.</u> **The following disciplines are related to the research of cancer research: immunology and cancer related group; virus and cancer related group; endocrine and cancer related group; fungi and cancer related group; Chronic inflammation related group; molecular biology and cancer related group; gene and cancer related group; environment and cancer related group. (See another article)**

The existing oncology talent, mostly for the radiotherapy and chemotherapy, education must be launched to capture the cancer total attack to train the personnel, apply their knowledge. Education is used for the construction of innovative countries, apply their knowledge, and it can be innovative results.

7. The past and the future of oncology development

(1) ***twice leaps which treatment of malignant tumors appeared in the two centuries***

Looking back over the past 100 years, human being is contempt by cancer, so far the formation of cancer is still the lack of the most essential understanding, the normal cell proliferation is subject to what factors control, and how they lost control of proliferation and become malignant cells.

In the last two centuries, the treatment of malignant tumors has experienced two leaps:

The first was in 1890 Halstad proposed the concept of tumor radicalization.

The second time was in the 1970s. Fish integrated chemotherapy into radical surgery (adjuvant chemotherapy or neoadjuvant chemotherapy).

Since then, malignant tumor treatment has been faltering

Fish is a systemic intravenous route. After half a century, it has not been able to reduce mortality, and it has not stopped recurrence, metastasis, and mortality.

Now we question and reform the traditional doctrine of the traditional method of administration, innovative opinions, changed to target organ intravascular administration, combined with the establishment of XZ-C comprehensive treatment concept and XZ-C immunomodulation therapy (ie immunochemotherapy), it will probably help to push the current status quo.

(2) President Nixon issued the Anti-Cancer Declaration in 1971 and filed an anti-cancer slogan in his joint speech.

In 1971 the United States Congress passed a "National Cancer Regulations", and by President Nixon issued "anti-cancer declaration", then put a considerable human and financial resources, with a view to overcome cancer in one fell swoop.

In December 1971, President Richard Nixon presented the anti-cancer slogan in the United Nations.

42 years have passed, and now Nixon has also been ancient, in cancer research it has also made many significant progress, such as the discovery of tumor suppressor genes, the advent of monoclonal antibodies, CT and magnetic resonance imaging, ultrasound and endoscopy and the improvement of various treatment methods of innovation.

However, in the current 20 years of the 21st century, the first 10 years, the largest human threats of lung cancer, colon cancer and other mortality rate is still basically the same as 50 years ago, cancer deaths are still the first cause of death of urban and rural residents in China.

__So the experts in medicine, biology and related disciplines began to reflect, most scientists believe that the prevention and treatment of the tumor should start from the most basic issues, that is, from the nature of cancer cells, pathogenesis, cancer cell metabolic characteristics and signal transduction to understand the cancer "Lushan__ *true face", only as this, it is to have the most effective prevention and treatment of cancer.*

To carry out interdisciplinary research, to promote basic research and clinical research cooperation, attention to clinical research.

It must be carried out clinical basic research and if there is no breakthrough in basic research, the clinical efficacy is difficult to improve.

(3) In 1982, Oldham founded *the theory of biological response regulation, on the basis of which he proposed in 1984, the fourth mode of cancer treatment (four modatity of cancer treatment) biological therapy. According to the theory of biological response, under normal circumstances, tumor and body defense are in a dynamic balance between the occurrence of tumor and even invasion, metastasis, is entirely caused by this dynamic imbalance. The state of the imbalance has been artificially adjusted to the normal level, you can control the growth of the tumor and make it subside.*

Biotherapy is to adjust this biological response by supplementing, inducing, or activating the cellular viable, biological, and / or cytokines that are inherent in the inherent bioreaction regulatory system.

Biological therapy is different from the previous three other treatment modes, namely, surgery, radiation therapy and chemotherapy to directly attack the tumor as the goal. *The scope of biotherapy is significantly beyond the traditional concept of immunotherapy, because the dynamic balance between the body and the tumor is not limited to the immune response, but also related to a variety of tumor-related regulatory genes and cytokines.*

Biological response regulator (BRM) has opened up a new field of tumor biotherapy, at present, BRM is as the fourth program of the tumor by the medical profession attention.

(4) As cancer patients become more and more, the incidence rate is rising, the mortality rate is high, recognizing that cancer should not only pay attention to treatment, but also pay attention to prevention, to prevent the source. The research aims should focus on the prevention and treatment of the whole process of cancer occurrence and development.

Xu Ze Put forward "strategic outlets and suggestions for conquering cancer." in "New Concepts and New Methods for Cancer Treatment" published in October.

In June 2013 XZ-C also proposed " the general idea and design to overcome the cancer and launch the total attack " in an attempt to reduce the incidence of cancer, reduce mortality, improve the cure rate, prolong survival.

The total attack that is the three carriages of prevention of cancer + control cancer + cancer treatment go hand in hand

The prevention of cancer:

By building a "two-oriented society" and building a well-off society, "catch-up scientific research" can achieve Class I prevention of cancer.

Control cancer:

Through the "three early" clinic, precancerous lesions were treated and screened.

Treatment of cancer:

surgery + immune regulation + biological therapy + differentiation induction therapy + integrated traditional Chinese and Western medicine treatment are as the main methods and the radiotherapy and chemotherapy are as a supplement.

Recent goals:

Suppress the momentum of cancer mania development, reduce its incidence rate, and gradually improve the cure rate, gradually realizing three 1/3.

- **One third of cancer can be prevented**
- **One third of cancer can be cured by early treatment**
- **One-third of patients can relieve pain through effective treatment**

To be victory over cancer, where is the road?

How do I see cancer?

The author (XU ZE) thinks of :

The road is in the scientific research, the road is the scientific research of the prevention and treatment of cancer;

The road is the scientific experimental research of exploring he cause of cancer, pathogenesis, pathophysiology;

The road is in the scientific experimental research of the whole process of the occurrence and development of cancer;

The road is the study of the reform and development of traditional therapy;

The road is to carry out multidisciplinary research, the formation of the relevant specialist group, special in-depth basis and clinical disciplines;

The road is the study of animal experimental research and basic and clinical research of cancer metastasis, recurrence prevention and treatment ;

The road is the study on the diagnosis and treatment techology of "three early" and precancerous lesions.

Through the scientific research of cancer prevention and treatment, mankind will overcome cancer and ultimately will overcome cancer.

Create the cancer prevention and treatment hospital during the whole process of cancer occurrence and development

(Global Demonstration of Cancer Prevention and Treatment Hospital)

The envisage and feasibility o build Wuhan anti-cancer hospital throughout the prevention and treatment

----- Explain the necessity and feasibility of establishing a full-scale hospital for prevention and treatment

At present, cancer has become a major disease that seriously threatens human health, and its incidence is increasing at an annual rate of 3% to 5%. The number of morbidity and deaths increased by 24.7% and 19.2% respectively compared with 10 years ago. The traditional three major treatment methods have been nearly 100 years old, and the mortality rate of cancer patients is still the first. What should I do? How should the road go? It is worthwhile for us to review, reflect, analyze and summarize the positive and negative experiences and lessons of success and failure and to think about why traditional therapy does not significantly reduce mortality, why not control recurrence and metastasis? What problems exist in traditional therapy and traditional concepts should be studied in depth.

Where is the cancer road?

How to overcome cancer?

The author believes that the road is in scientific research, the road is in the scientific research on cancer prevention and treatment, and the road is scientific research in the whole process of studying cancer occurrence and development.

The road is in the study of the reform, promotion and development of traditional therapy, and the road in the "three early".

Through scientific research on cancer prevention and treatment, human beings will surely overcome cancer, and will eventually overcome cancer.

It is necessary to set up a whole-course prevention and treatment hospital for cancer, and carry out medical practice and practical work for prevention and treatment of the whole process. Under the guidance of the scientific concept of development, with the vision of development, with the spirit of innovation, gaze forward, face the future, develop medicine, develop cancer prevention and treatment medicine in practice, practice real knowledge, and work hard to achieve the goal of conquering cancer.

1. The urgent need of the current oncology discipline is to carry out the cancer scientific research

(1) It must be aware of the current problems of oncology

① the basic problem is that the three traditional treatment has been applied for nearly a hundred years, the cancer mortality rate is still the first urban and rural areas. What should we do? It is should be analyzed, reflected and researched.

② postoperative recurrence is still very serious; the patients and their families are afraid of recurrence; some patients fears or are anxious for all day long after surgery. How should the surgeon prevent recurrence, prevent postoperative metastasis? It is to deserve our study.

③ metastasis is the core of cancer, is the key to survival, everyone is afraid of cancer metastasis. How effective anti-cancer metastasis, control cancer cell metastasis? should it be carried out basic and clinical research?

④ It must recognize the status of the existence of tumor disciplines. what are the problems? how can it be done? Although cancer treatment has been more than a century, it has now entered the second decade of the 21st century, but "oncology" is still the most backward of the current medical disciplines, why? It is because the etiology, pathogenesis, pathophysiology of "oncology" are not yet clear. Oncology of the scientific research is a virgin land and need to have a lot of basic scientific research and clinical basic research. Conducting cancer science research is an urgent need for current oncology disciplines.

⑤ Although countries invest a lot of money for the treatment of cancer patients, although the traditional three treatment for nearly a hundred years, but the cancer mortality rate is still the first reason for the death of urban and rural residents in China, the main reasons are the following:

A. the etiology of cancer is not entirely clear, the pathogenesis of cancer cell metastasis mechanism is still lack of understanding.

B. it is lack of adequate understanding of the complex biological behavior of cancer.

C. the treatment program is still quite blind.

D. the diagnostic means are behind, once found, that is late, so the result of the treatment is poor.

E. many large hospitals have not established a laboratory, can not carry out the basic research of cancer, anti-cancer metastasis, recurrence, must be involved in cancer animal model of basic research, because if no basic research breakthrough, the clinical efficacy is difficult to improve.

(2) It must be aware of the current problems of treatment

① chemotherapy needs to be further research and improvement

Whether postoperative adjuvant chemotherapy prevents recurrence, whether it prevents metastasis, and how it can help prevent postoperative recurrence and metastasis or not are worthy of our study, we should come up with their own data and experience to conduct further research and refinement.

Through the clinical medical practice case review, analysis, and reflection, it was found:

A. some patients with adjuvant chemotherapy failed to prevent recurrence;

B. some patients postoperative adjuvant chemotherapy failed to prevent metastasis;

C. some patients postoperative adjuvant chemotherapy to promote immune failure.

Through the review, analysis, and reflection of the current status of tumor chemotherapy in China, it was found:

A. traditional chemotherapy to suppress immune function, inhibition of bone marrow hematopoietic function, immune decline can promote tumor development.

B. white blood cell (WBC) reduction is one of the common toxicity of chemotherapy, WBC decline can lead to serious infection → a large number of antibiotics → double infection (fungal infection) → immune failure.

C. the traditional chemotherapy damage to the host, because the chemotherapy cell poison as a "double-edged sword", that is, killing cells and kill normal cells (chemotherapy drugs about 99.6%, kill normal cells, especially bone marrow hematopoietic cells and immune cells, only about 0.4% Drug cancer cells)

D. the traditional intravenous chemotherapy for intermittent treatment, intermittent cannot be treated, that is, there is the role of killing cancer cells only 3-5 days of intravenous administration, then no killing cancer cells (Figure 1), it is only a short time to kill (3-5), can not once and for all, after 3-5 days the cancer cells continue to proliferate, split (Figure 2), so it can only alleviate in a short time.

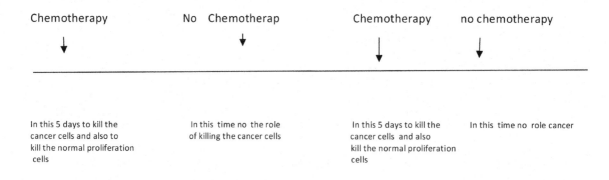

Figure 1 time to kill cancer cells

E. the traditional therapy target only focus on chemotherapy can kill cancer cells, while ignoring the host itself on cancer resistance and control, because the tumor occurs, the development depends on the level of host immune function and the biological characteristics of the tumor itself, that decision The biological characteristics of the tumor cells and the host of the constraints on the two factors than the potential, if the balance is controlled, if the two imbalance is progress.

Traditional radiotherapy and chemotherapy are to promote the decline in immune function, it is possible to make the two more unbalanced.

F. *whether is the solid tumor (stomach, colorectal, liver, gallbladder, pancreas, spleen, abdominal, pelvic and other tumors) systemic intravenous chemotherapy route scientific and reasonable or not? It should be questioned.*

a. This route of administration, through the heart pump to chemotherapy cells to the body distribution of toxic drugs, killing the body organs of the organs, it is unreasonable.

Now many solid malignancies, postoperative adjuvant chemotherapy were used intravenous intravenous infusion, the elbow vein infusion → superior vena cava → right heart → through the pulmonary artery into the lungs → via the pulmonary vein into the left heart → through the aortic flow distribution in the body The (About 0.4%), and the vast majority (about 99.6%) of the chemotherapy cells are distributed in the body organs and kill normal cells, especially immune cells, bone marrow hematopoietic cells, resulting in The patient was severely damaged, serious side effects, and the solid foci did not play a significant role. Therefore, the above-mentioned solid tumor intravenous chemotherapy route of administration is unreasonable, unscientific, the cytotoxic system is distributed, is damaged in the patient.

b. This route of administration can not be directly reached the portal vein system, vena cava system and the portal vein system is generally not connected by the superior vena cava is difficult to reach the portal vein.

Chemotherapy is to use cytotoxic cancer cells, must first study clear where the cancer cells are ? it is to be targeted, clear objectives. Along the line of cancer cell line transfer, the cancer cells to track and kill, and along the tumor vein flow, chemotherapy drugs can follow this path to kill the cancer cells are being transferred. So, stomach, colorectal, liver, gallbladder, pancreas, spleen, abdomen and other cancer cells in there? It is mainly in the hepatic portal vein system. But the vena cava system and the portal vein system is generally not connected by the elbow vein → vena cava route of administration can not enter the portal vein system, so the abdominal tumor of the systemic intravenous chemotherapy route of administration is unreasonable, unscientific, Detrimental to the patient. It is because it cannot enter the portal vein system where cancer cells exist.

For half a century, tens of thousands of cancer patients around the world have suffered from the huge pain of widespread killing of normal cells by chemotherapy. Clinicians should seriously think, analyze, reflect, evaluate. For the solid tumor should not be administered by the elbow vein, but should try to target the tube tube intravascular administration, should try to correct the current irrational route of administration, and to reform, innovation and development.

③ the current chemotherapy is often a certain blindness, postoperative adjuvant chemotherapy, the surgical specimens were not for cancer cell culture, and thus can not be the patient's cancer chemotherapy drug susceptibility test. The current courtyard alone experience patients with blind chemotherapy. It has a chemotherapy and do not know whether to kill cancer cells and it can only be said to have completed a chemotherapy work. It may be beneficial to some patients, but may be harmful to a considerable number of patients, if the patient is resistant to the drug, it is not only beneficial, but harmful.

(3) the main contradiction of current chemotherapy

So far, the purpose of tumor chemotherapy is still mainly to kill cancer cells, the drugs used are mostly cytotoxic, no selectivity, regardless of cancer cells or normal cells will be damaged. Through the case review, analysis, reflection, I realized that the existence of the following several major contradictions in chemotherapy.

① the contradiction between the chemotherapeutic drug poison and the damaged host

The purpose of the treatment of cancer is to eliminate the tumor, to protect the body, to restore health, and the current chemotherapy is to kill both the tumor and the normal cells and hurt the host and lose everything.

② persistent and intermittent contradictions

Cancer cells continue to split, and the contradiction between intermittent chemotherapy, cancer cell proliferation and division of cell cycle proliferation is continuous, and because of its inhibition of bone marrow hematopoietic function and peripheral white blood cells, chemotherapy drugs can only be used intermittently; there is a contradiction between cell division and intermittent chemotherapy. Even in the 3-5 days of chemotherapy to kill most of the cancer cells, but after a few days, the efficacy disappeared, the remaining cancer stem cells will continue to split, proliferation, cloning, recurrence, metastasis. Therefore, simply kill cancer cells do not meet the biological characteristics of cancer cells and biological behavior.

③ The contradiction of rising immune function and falling immune function

The use of chemotherapy drugs tends to reduce the immune function of patients, and there is a contradiction with cancer treatment must improve the immune function. Chemotherapy drugs are leading to decreased immune function; the longer the course of treatment, the more the decline in immune function, or even lose immune surveillance, cancer cells spread further.

(4) Radiotherapy need to be further studied and improved

Radiotherapy is for local treatment and the transfer is systemic problems. How to play its role in anti-metastatic therapy? how to protect the patient's organs from nuclear radiation damage? It is to be further studied and improved.

(5)The "radical surgery" design need to be further studied and improved to reduce postoperative recurrence and metastasis. Since it is "radical surgery", why does not it achieve the purpose of radical treatment? Since doing lymph node dissection, why transfer? These are required for further study. How to reduce the intraoperative tumor-free technology? how to reduce and to prevent intraoperative cancer cell shedding? how to reduce the intraoperative promotion of cancer cell metastasis? how to reduce the spread from the tumor vein? All of these are things which clinicians should pay attention to the problems in the practices. Surgical operation should be light, stable and accurate. Surgery is the primary methods to prevent the transfer, to prevent postoperative recurrence and metastasis and it must be done from the surgery and should prevent the operation of cancer cells to protect the shedding, planting, spread.

2, the existing problems of the current building tumor hospital model

(1) the current status of the tumor hospital

① background and sub-division

1. General provincial tumor hospital with tumor surgery, cancer gynecology, oncology, radiotherapy, chemotherapy, comprehensive … … and other subjects

2. Department of Oncology Hospital and the top three hospital of the tumor only have oncology, radiotherapy, chemotherapy, comprehensive … … and other subjects

3. Surgical cancer surgery treatment is performed in surgery

4. Gynecological cancer surgery treatments are in gynecology

5. Orthopedic cancer surgery treatment are in orthopedics

6. ENT cancer treatments are in the ENT

② tasks and objects

The task is mainly treatment, the object is mainly in the late, transfer, relapse of patients with poor efficacy.

③ treatment: mainly kill cancer cells

Radiotherapy, chemotherapy, chemotherapy + radiotherapy

④ treatment results: the mortality rate is still the first, the incidence is still rising

(2) The existence problems of the hospital model

① focus on the focus of treatment, for the late, metastasis, recurrence of advanced cancer patients with poor efficacy, exhausted human and financial resources, and failed to achieve lower mortality, improve the cure rate, reduce morbidity.

② only treatment, or heavy treatment with light defense, the more treatment and the more patients.

③ ignored the commitment to "three early", early detection, early diagnosis, early treatment. The Early patients have the good curative effect and the high cure rate.

④ ignore the precancerous state, precancerous lesions of the treatment

⑤ ignored the prevention

(3) It should be reformed, innovated and developed for the problems existing in the unification mode

① solve the hospital model, and gradually solve the prevention and treatment at the same attention and the focus shifted to the left.

To solve the problem of prevention and treatment, prevention and control strategy, prevention and treatment strategy, the goal is to reduce morbidity, reduce mortality and improve the cure rate.

In order to improve the therapeutic effect, improve the cure rate and reduce the mortality rate, we must pay attention to the above: "it must understand the current problems in the treatment", to further study and improve, for the above problems to be reform, innovation and development. So as to improve the quality of medical care, reduce mortality and improve the cure rate.

③ in order to control cancer → fight cancer → capture cancer, the goal must be to reduce morbidity, reduce mortality, improve the cure rate, it should be both treatment and control. Building hospitals should be the hospital with cancer prevention and treatment at the same attention .

Building journals should be a magazine on tumor prevention and control, and should be both important for prevention and treatment. Both medical and educational and scientific research must be both important for prevention and control.

Medical school teaching work curriculum must be the prevention and treatment at the same level.

Scientific research project set up must be both the prevention and treatment at the same level.

Tumor and Environmental Science and Life Sciences and Ecological Sciences must be multidisciplinary to infiltrate, create new disciplines, discipline disciplines, and develop new industries.

So, it will be to overcome cancer → conquest cancer → capture cancer, will improve cancer prevention, control, treatment .

3. The status quo of the current incidence of cancer in China

The current cancer has become a major threat to human health, the main disease, the incidence of an average annual rate of 3% -5% increase. According to the National Cancer Registration Center released the "2012 China Cancer Registration Annual Report." New cases of cancer each year are about 312 million cases, an average of 8550 per day, the country every minute there are six people diagnosed with cancer.

Malignant tumor disease rate of 35 to 39 years of age were 87.07 / 10 million.

In 40 to 44 years old age it was 154.53 / 10 million.

In More than 50 years of age it accounted for more than 80% of the total incidence of the disease.

More than 1% of the incidence of cancer over 60 years of age.

In 80 years of age it is to reach the peak.

National cancer mortality rate was 180.54 / 10 million, each year due to cancer deaths it is 2.7 million cases. The probability of cancer deaths among Chinese residents is 13%, that is, one in every seven to eight people is killed by cancer. Tumor mortality was higher in men than in women, 1.68: 1.

From the disease, the first place in the national malignant tumor is lung cancer, followed by gastric cancer, colorectal cancer, liver cancer and esophageal cancer. **Ranking first in the national malignant tumor is still lung cancer, followed by liver cancer, stomach cancer, esophageal cancer and colorectal cancer. The highest mortality rate, both men and women are lung cancer**.

Although cancer treatment has been going on for more than a century, it has entered the second decade of the 21st century, Statistics from the Beijing Municipal Health Bureau show that In 2010, lung cancer ranked first in the incidence of male malignancies in Beijing's registered population, ranking second in women, second only to breast cancer. From 2001 to 2010, the incidence of lung cancer in the city increased by 56%. One-fifth of all new cancers in the city are lung cancer patients.

The incidence of lung cancer in urban population in China is close to that of developed countries. Wei Shaozhong, director of the Hubei Cancer Center, introduced in 2009 there were 12,590 registered cancer patients in Wuhan.

There were 6961 deaths, which was equivalent to 1049 people with cancer per month and 580 people died of cancer.

Cancer incidence in Wuhan from 2003 to 2009 increased from 165.82/100,000 to 257.89/100,000 and increased year after year, and is consistent with the national situation, the incidence and mortality of lung cancer in Wuhan is high. By gender, women have a high rate of breast cancer.

The first five cancers in male in Wuhan are lung cancer, liver cancer, colorectal cancer, gastric cancer, urogenital cancer, the first five women is breast cancer, lung cancer, reproductive system cancer, colon cancer, gastric cancer.

The incidence of female breast cancer is high, but the mortality rate is much lower than lung cancer, indicating early diagnosis and treatment of breast cancer early results. As early as early detection, early treatment, it can achieve better treatment, and even cured.

4, how can it be to reduce the incidence of cancer? How can we improve cancer cure rate?

It must be the prevention of the cancer and control of the cancer and treatment of cancer and change the hospital building mode.

So how to prevent it? How to control? How to cure?

How to improve the cure rate?

——*The way out for cancer treatment is "three early"*

How to reduce the incidence rate? How to reduce morbidity?

——The way to fight cancer is prevention

At present, the treatment of cancer in each tumor hospital or oncology is mainly concentrated in the middle and late stages, and the treatment effect is poor.

(1), how to improve cancer cure rate? the way-out of Cancer treatment is in the "three early"

Cancer's production and growth will go through stage of susceptibility, precancerous lesion and invasive stage. All the present tumor hospitals or tumor departments mainly focus on the cancer treatment in middle or advanced stage. The Therapeutic effects are poor. If patients in middle or advanced stage can accept surgical operation, then they will be treated surgically. But if not, they will only receive palliative treatment. Therefore, cancer treatment lies in "early detection, early diagnosis and early treatment". Generally, patients in the early stage will get a better therapeutic effect. The increase of therapeutic effect will certainly reduce the fatality rate of cancer. Consequently, we must put much emphasis on the study of early-stage diagnostic and therapeutic methods, and on the treatment of precancerous lesion for lessening medium-term or terminal patients in the invasive stage.

stage of susceptibility	precancerous lesion	early stage	no metastasis	have metastasized	
				local position	amphi position

①   ②   ③   ④   ⑤   ⑥

① Cancer prevention

② Outpatient service of "three kinds of earliness"

③ Surgical operation

④ Place surgical operation first, radiotherapy, chemotherapy and biological TCM second

⑤ Possible to undergo surgical operation

⑥ To give treatment as carcinomatous metastasis

If patients have been treated well in the stage of precancerous lesion or early stage, then the number of patients in middle or advanced stage of invasion and metastasis will fall off. Thus, the cancer incidence rate will also decline. Therefore, we hold that the present tumor hospitals in various places mainly focus on the cancer treatment in middle or advanced stage. Even though the therapeutic result is effective, it can only bring the reduction of cancer mortality rate. But if ignoring the stage of susceptibility, precancerous lesion or early stage, it will be impossible to reduce the cancer incidence rate. Therefore, we must put much emphasis on the whole process of cancer production and growth. After all this is the real global change of strategic importance.

The writer has engaged in surgical oncology for over sixty years. More and more patients suffer from cancer, and the cancer incidence rate also rises. The writer deeply feels that people should emphasize not only therapy but also prevention. Only in this way could the cancer be killed in the source. Cancer treatment lies in "three kinds of earliness" (early detection, early diagnosis and early treatment); anti-cancer method lies in prevention.

As stated above, the strategic center of gravity of tumor treatment and prevention moves forward. There are two aspects in its meaning. One is to prevent cancer by changing life style and improving environmental pollution; the other is to cure precancerous lesion for inhibiting cancer's development to the invasion stage, middle stage or advanced stage.

In 1990, our institute's specialist out-patient department of tumor surgery once opened the outpatient service of "three kinds of earliness" to carry out various endoscopies and biopsies, through which have found many atypical hyperplasia of stomach, intestinal metaplasia, atrophic gastritis and hyperplasia of mammary glands, etc. These "precancerous lesions" are difficult to treat. Then how to handle these precancerous lesions or precancerous conditions so as to prevent their cancerations urgently needs clinical researches to look for better treatment methods.

(2). It should pay attention to the study of the diagnosis and treatment technology from the basic and clinical aspects for the precancerous lesions

"Three kinds of earliness" is the key to cancer treatment. While how to handle precancerous lesion is the key stage for cancer prevention and treatment.

The present cancer diagnosis mainly depends on image examinations of type-B ultrasonic, CT and MRI. But as soon as the cancer comes to light, it has reached the middle or advanced stage. Many patients have lost the chance of radical excision. Although the complex treatment has been done, the therapeutic effects are still poor. If the cancer is in the early stage or belongs to the carcinoma in situ, then the curative effect of operation will be better and the cancer can be cured. Therefore, the cancer treatment should strive for "three kinds of earliness", which refers to early detection, early diagnosis and early treatment.

Because cancer's pathogenic factors are not very clear, the primary prevention is still quite difficult.

Studies in recent years indicate that malignant tumor rarely has a direct carcinomatous change in normal tissues. Before the occurrence of tumor in clinical diagnosis, cancer often goes through quite a long evolution stage, which is the stage of precancerous lesion. Early identification and control of these precancerous lesions will bring positive significances for the secondary prevention of cancer.

What is precancerous lesion? The precancerous lesion is a histopathology concept, which refers to a kind of tissues with the dysplasia of cells. Precancerous lesion has the potential to become cancerous. If there is no cure in a long period, precancerous lesion will evolve into cancer. In other words, precancerous lesion just has the possibility of changing into cancer. But not all the precancerous lesions will eventually become cancer. Through proper treatments, precancerous lesions may return to their normal states or have a spontaneous regression.

Canceration is a developing process with several stages. There is a stage of precancerous lesion between normal cells and cancer. It is a slow process from precancerous lesion evolving into cancer, which needs many years or even more than ten years. The length of canceration course is closely related to the strength of carcinogenic factors, individual susceptibility and immunologic function. Therefore, the study of precancerous lesion is of great importance to cancer's prevention and control.

(3) More than one third of the cancer can be prevented

The tumor formation is a long process with several factors and stages. Precancerous lesion in the promotion stage is of reversibility, so cancer is preventable.

Multi-factor, multi-step and multi-stage characteristics of tumor onset:

The generation and growth of tumor can be roughly divided into several stages of initiation, promotion, metastasis and others. Cellular canceration induced by chemical carcinogen is a multistage process. The chemical carcinogenesis process of Experimental animals and the generating process of human tumors (such as colon cancer) have a series of changes, which are hyperplasia → pathological changes → benign tumor → malignant tumor → tumor metastasis, etc. The whole change process is complicated with multiple stages of initiation, promotion and evolution, etc. It often takes a long cytometaplasia time to change from normal cells to the tumor that can be detected clinically, which is a long cumulative process.

(1) Two-stage theory of tumor formation:

In 1942, Beremblum carried out the experimental study of mouse's skin canceration induction, in which he used benzoapyrene to treat mice's skins for about one year, and only three out of one hundred and two mice suffered from skin tumors. If mice's skins were treated with benzoapyrene for several months and then treated with the tumor promoter-croton oil, thirty-six out of eighty-three mice suffered from skin cancers, whose incidence rate was ten times higher than that of using benzoapyrene alone. If mice's skins were first treated with croton oil for several months and then treated with a carcinogenic substance, there would be no induced tumor. If mice's skins were only treated with croton oil for a long time, whose incidence rate of tumor would be lower than that of using benzoapyrene alone (1/106).

On the basis of this study results, Beremblum and Subik have proposed that cancerous process contains two different but intimate stages. **One is a specific provocation stage.** Small dosages of carcinogenic substance induce normal cells to become potential cancer cells. The other is **nonspecific promoting stage.** Potential cancer cells are further promoted to suffer from mutation and evolve into tumor under the action of tumor promoters, such as croton oil and others.

People hold that provocation process refers to the process that normal cells change into potential cancer cells under the action of carcinogenic substances. The time of promoting process is fairly short and generally irreversible. While promoting process is the process that potential cancer cells change into cancer cells under the action of tumor promoters. The early promoting stage is reversible but the late stage is irreversible.

Carcinogenic substance is a kind of mutagen, which plays a decisive role in canceration process. While cancer promoters do not have the mutagenicity, which can only promote potential cancer cells to have a further proliferation change and gradually evolve into cancer cells. During these two processes of provocation and promoting stages, induced cells grow out of control, escape from the host's immune surveillance, gradually form tumor cells with malignant phenotype and then evolve into tumor cells with infiltration and metastasis. This theory recognizes that tumor generation is quite a long process (months, years and even more than ten years) and will be impossible through a single factor or stage, *which is very important to cancer prevention and control. It prompts that people have enough time to build up cancer-fighting ability, strengthen immunity, change life style and improve environmental pollution to prevent cancer. Intervention measures should be emphasized to tackle the reversible stage of cancer promoting.*

(4) How to reduce the incidence of cancer? - The way out for cancer is prevention

For almost half a century, human spectrum of disease has undergone a drastic change. Most communicable diseases have been effectively controlled. Chronic diseases, such as cardiovascular diseases and malignant tumors have been the most serious diseases threatening human health.

Cancer has become the most serious public health problem in the world. Compared with other chronic diseases, cancer's prevention and control face a greater challenge.

Over the last thirty years, the fatality rate of cancer in China is on an obvious rise, which has occupied the number one in causes of death of urban and rural residents. On average, one out of every four deceased persons dies from cancer.

Cancer not only seriously threatens human health but also causes the rapid rise of hospitalization costs. The direct costs of cancer treatment in China are about one hundred billion RMB every year, which makes patients and the whole society bear a huge economic burden.

Although each country inputs a large number of funds to treat cancer patients, the five-year survival rate of some common cancers has no obvious improvement in the recent twenty years. For instance, during the years from 1974 to 1990 in USA, the five-year survival rate of esophagus cancer only rose from 7% to 9%, stomach cancer from 16% to 19%, liver cancer from 3% to 6%, lung cancer from 12% to 15% and that of pancreatic cancer remained the same as 3%.

What's to be done? Anti-cancer method lies in prevention. Prevention and intervention is the most important thing in the field of public health.

As for the malignant cancer, prevention outweighs therapy. Worldwide tumor researchers have reached a consensus of adjusting public health resources and policies, shifting strategic focus from therapy to prevention, and carrying out positive and effective studies of pre-warning, early diagnosis and intervention to lower tumor incidence rate and raise curative rate.

According to the evidence provided by the World Health Organization's Cancer Report, as many as one third of cancers can be prevented. As long as governments, medical workers and the general public take positive actions, the focus of cancer prevention research will be shifted to prevention, and more than one third or even half of cancers can be prevented.

5. The road of how to overcome cancer is to study the establishment of hospital of prevention and treatment of cancer during the whole process of cancer occurrence and development and change the current building hospital mode which focuses on treatment and ignores defense

XU ZE provided on the strategic thinking, planning sketches, of the prevention and treatment of cancer during the whole process of occurrence and development ; how to overcome of cancer ? The road is to study the prevention and treatment of cancer during the whole process of cancer occurrence and development, practice a real knowledge, practice to product the results.

Xu ZE (Xu ZE) provided on the thought, strategy and program against cancer are shown in the following schematic drawing.

How to overcome cancer?

↓

Where is the way?

↓

Our thought, strategy and experience should be divided into three parts

↓

Before the formation of cancer——prevention part——anti- mutation

↓

Precancerous lesion with possible tendency of malignant change——intervention part

↓

The therapeutic part of primary cancer with the formation of focus and anti-metastasis

↓

Stage of preventing susceptibility   precancerous lesion   cancer and metastasis

a1   a2   a3 b1 b2 b3 b4

Primary lesion ———— Metastasis ——→

↓   Chemotherapy and radiotherapy   ↓

Surgical operation

↓   ①②③④⑤⑥ ①② ③④

c1   c2

a1. "Two-oriented society" contains essences and measures

a2. "Lift scientific research" makes plans and measures of cancer control

a3. Propaganda, education and study of popular science

b1. General investigation of physical examination

b2. Selective examination of high risk group

b3. Outpatient service of "early detection, early diagnosis and early treatment"

b4. Induced differentiation

c1. Improve free-tumor technique

c2. Prevent intraoperative implantation of cast-off cells

① with indication

② individuation

③ scientization

④ drug sensitive test

⑤ try to reduce untoward reaction

⑥ "intelligent resistance to cancer" of target administration

① targeted therapy

② anti-metastasis and anti-relapse therapies

③ BRM biological therapy

④ immunoregulation therapy

Figure. The diagram of the strategic thinking of prevention and treatment of cancer during the whole process of development and occurrence

I am going to apply for a new idea and a new approach to the occurrence and development of cancer, as shown in the plan diagram, according to my third book, "New Concepts and New Methods for the Treatment of Cancer", in Chapter 38, page 308 as the hospital of the prevention and treatment, unlike the current hospital mode is the invasion as the main.

This kind of innovative hospital mode is aimed at the prevention and treatment of the whole process of cancer occurrence and development. It is closely related to the clinical practice. In view of the existing problems and shortcomings of the traditional therapy, this paper puts forward a series of suggestions and innovation and development.

五

The basic design and feasibility of preparation of the envisage of the total attack and the science city for conquering cancer

--- is equivalent to the design of the overall framework with a Chinese characteristics of capturing cancer

Why is it put forward the general imagination and design of overcoming cancer ? How to attack? It should be a comprehensive planning and layout

1. Recognize the need to put forward the total attack

(1) in the research journey it is gradually to recognize the need to put forward the total attack

This initiative is a review, reflection, analysis, summary of successful experiences and lessons of failure in a large number of clinical practice cases of long-term cancer specialist out-patient clinics for more than 30 years, and progressively and slowly recognized and put forward. These acquaintances mainly appear in my three monographs, I recovered after a serious illness, quietly to hide in the small building for 18 years with solitary military alone war, went it alone, summed up their own experimental research and clinical validation information, has published three monographs, in the first monograph "new understanding and new model of cancer treatment" was published in 2001, which in the book it was put forward to a new understanding and in the international community it was first proposed "chemotherapy to be further research and improvement." At that time people are afraid to agree, but some patients and doctors have feelings. In 2002 when participating in the Barcelona International Medical Association Conference and reporting it, it received an excellent paper certificate.

The second monograph "new concepts and new methods of cancer metastasis therapy" was published in 2006 and was based on the first book on the basis of scientific research, the "target" of the cancer treatment was located in the anti-metastasis, indicating that the key of cancer treatment is anti-metastasis.

It was conducted a series of the experimental research and clinical basic research and clinical validation research of anti - cancer metastasis and recurrence, and rose to the theoretical innovation, and it was put forward the new idea and the methods of anti – metastasis. In April 2007 it was received the "three hundred" original book award issued by the People's Republic of China Press and Publication Administration.

The third monograph "new concept and new method of cancer treatment" was published in 2011, is based on the second monograph research results on the basis of forward development, the research objectives focused on the study of prevention and treatment during the whole process of cancer occurrence and development; it is close to connect with the clinical reality, aimed at the existence problems and shortcomings of traditional treatment of the current clinical practice, it was put forward the reform and innovation and research and development; it is realized that cancer prevention and treatment strategy must move forward, the way out of treatment of cancer is in the "three early" and in the prevention. The book was published in April 2013, and was published in Washington and sold in globe such as UK Europe and America.

I have been engaged in tumor surgery for 57 years, more and more patients, the incidence of cancer is also rising, high mortality rate, so I deeply appreciate that cancer should not only pay attention to treatment, but also pay attention to prevention, in order to stop at the source.

Three monographs are three different stages, three different levels of height, three different understandings. In the different levels of height there is the different scenery and there are the different understanding, different eyes; a mountain is higher than a mountain and a mountain has better scenery than a mountain. (This is just three books comparing with their own)

Therefore, after the third monograph, I put forward the task, mission, opportunity and challenge of anti-cancer research, under the guidance of the scientific concept of development, take the Chinese characteristics of anti-cancer metastasis research and innovation, put forward the strategic thinking and suggestions of conquering cancer and put forward the need for total attack.

Under the situation of the current high incidence of cancer and high mortality rate it is realized the need to launch a total attack.

People have been fighting cancer for hundreds of years, but so far cancer is still rampant in the crowd and it is the effectiveness of the emblem and the incidence is still rising and the mortality rate is high.

According to statistics in 1995, the world's annual new cancer is 7 million people, the number of deaths each year is 500 million people. In China's cancer in 1996 the number is 1.8 million, the death toll is 1.28 million. In terms of mortality, the tumor is at the head of the disease and becomes the most serious disease that threatens human health.

"2012 China Cancer Registration Annual Report", the annual new cancer fell to 312 million cases, the average daily 8550 people, in the country every minute there are 6 people diagnosed with cancer. The current cancer is the first cause of the death of urban and rural residents in China, and every one of the seven deaths is cancer.

The current cancer has become a serious threat to human health and the main disease; the incidence of an average annual rate increases by 3% -5% of the incidence rate, the more treatment and the more patients, the mortality rate is high. People should not do nothing, humans should not sit still, I think we should put forward the general idea of conception and basic design of conquering cancer and it is the time to "declared war on cancer" and it should launch the total attack.

(2) To recognize the problems and drawbacks of radiotherapy and chemotherapy and it is difficult to rely on them to conquering cancer, under this condition it is to raise the need to launch a general attack

① **Review of the traditional three therapies in the century and historical evaluation**

Three treatments of Cancer traditional therapy: surgical treatment, radiotherapy, chemotherapy have been for nearly a hundred years, how are the results of its treatment? It should be reviewed and evaluated about the efficacy for a century, from theory to practice, to the efficacy. Can it be relied on three major treatments to conquer cancer in the future? How is its prospects assessment ? The evaluation criteria are: reduce morbidity, reduce mortality, prolong survival, improve quality of life, reduce complications.

We should calm down, sort out, analyze data, review, reflect, and summarize the experiences and lessons of both positive and negative aspects of success and failure. What are the results? What are the lessons? Has the patient benefited? Whether it has prolonged life and eased the pain: the successful experience should be carefully analyzed, the lessons learned from failure should be carefully summed up, the problems existing should be identified, and the experience and lessons learned. Think about why traditional treatments do not significantly reduce mortality? It should think about why traditional therapy does not control recurrence and metastasis? It should be considered why the three major treatments have been nearly a hundred years old. Is the cancer death rate still the first death of our city and township residents?

I have been in Tongji Medical College for 62 years, and I have been working in cancer surgery for 57 years. Experienced and witnessed the traditional three major treatments for half a century. Deeply think about how to evaluate the efficacy of the century.

What is the treatment of cancer patients? It is often considered to be: the patient's survival period is long, good quality of life, symptoms improved, fewer complications.

The three major means of the traditional treatment of cancer has made a brilliant contribution to human anti-cancer business. However, until the first two decades of the 21st century, cancer is still rampant, the more treatment and the more patients, the incidence of cancer continues to rise, high mortality, remains the first cause of urban and rural deaths in China.

Although the patient has undergone regular, systemic radiotherapy and / or chemotherapy after surgery, it has not been able to prevent the recurrence of cancer cells. Why traditional treatment did not significantly reduce mortality? Does it suggest that traditional therapies do not meet the biological characteristics of cancer cells? What is the problem with traditional radiotherapy and chemotherapy? What is the traditional concept of cancer therapies? What is theoretically or conceptual problem? How to correct its shortcomings on the concept or understanding so that it becomes the more perfect?

Through the review and analysis and evaluation and reflection of clinical practice cases and postoperative adjuvant chemotherapy cases, it was found that there are problems:

(1) in some patients the postoperative adjuvant chemotherapy failed to prevent recurrence;

(2) in some patients the postoperative adjuvant chemotherapy failed to prevent metastasis;

(3) in some patients the chemotherapy promotes immune failure.

From the clinical practice of case to analysis and reflect why the postoperative chemotherapy failed to prevent cancer recurrence, metastasis?

From the role of chemotherapy drugs in the cancer cell cycle to analyze and reflect; from the chemical drugs to suppress the overall immune function to analyze and reflect; from the drug resistance of chemotherapy to analyze and to reflect it was found:

(1) For the current chemotherapy there are some important errors;

(2) the current chemotherapy exists to a major contradiction.

Through the review, analysis, evaluation, reflection of the clinical medical practice case it was found the following problems:

"Analysis, evaluation and questioning of systemic intravenous chemotherapy for solid tumors"; (see another article)

"Review, analysis and commentary on the three major treatments for cancer"; (see another article)

"Chemotherapy needs to be further research and improvement." (See another article)

Update thinking, update awareness

Through the review and analysis and evaluation and self-reflection of 7 years of experimental experiments and 30 years of specialist outpatient clinics on more than 6,000 cases of diagnosis and treatment, it is summed up the success and failure of both positive and negative experience and lessons and it was thought of why the traditional therapy did not significantly reduce the death Rate? why did not it control relapse and transfer? What are the questions of the traditional concept of traditional therapy? So I gradually realize that the current cancer traditional therapies may still have some important errors. *For example:*

1) *the traditional chemotherapy suppresses the immune function and inhibit the bone marrow hematopoietic function;*

2) *the conventional intravenous chemotherapy is the intermittent treatment; in the intermittent period cancer can not be treated and intermittent cancer cells continue to proliferate and divide;*

3) *traditional therapy damage the host, because the chemotherapy cell poison for the "double-edged sword", both kill cancer cells and kill normal cells;*

4) *traditional therapy goal only focuses on that chemotherapy can kill cancer cells, while ignoring the host itself on cancer resistance and control because the occurrence and development of the tumor depends on the level of host immune function and the biological characteristics of the tumor itself, that is determined by The biological characteristics of tumor cells and the host of the constraints on the impact of the two potential, if it is the balance, cancer is controlled; if the two are imbalance, cancer is progress. Traditional radiotherapy and chemotherapy are to promote the decline in immune function and it may make the two more potential imbalance;*

5) *The traditional therapy damages the central immune organs, cancer Thymus has been inhibited, and chemotherapy inhibits bone marrow, as "snow plus frogs or worse". So that the entire central immune organs were damaged and failed to effectively protect;*

6) *The traditional therapy is injury therapy and has a certain blow to the the entire central immune organs which can not be effectively protected;*

7) *Traditional therapy neglects the anti-cancer ability of the human body itself, ignores the role of anticancer cells (NK cell population, K cell population, LAK cell population, macrophage population, TK cell population) in the host cancer system and ignores the role of the host of the anti-cancer cytokine system IFN, IL-2, TNF, LT and ignores the role of the host of the tumor suppressor gene and tumor suppressor gene (the human body has oncogenes and tumor suppressor genes, but also cancer metastasis gene and tumor suppressor gene) and ignores the role of the neurohumoral system and endocrine hormone system in the body and ignores the role of anti-cancer agencies and their influencing factors in the human body, as well as its role of the regulation, balance and stabilization of the host mechanism itself and ignores the inherent factors of the human body's anti-cancer activity, Blindly kill cancer cellsy kill cancer cells;*

8) *Traditional therapy goal is relatively simple, just kill cancer cells. And it is not consistent with the actual situation of the biological characteristics of cancer now known such as cancer cell invasion behavior; the metastasis is involved in the multiple steps; the incentives factors of the relapse can be the latent months or years and then have recurrence. It has been recognized*

that antineoplastic agents are not necessarily resistant to metastasis and the anti-metastatic drugs are not necessarily anti-tumor.

How to do? Both the above problems should be further research, and conduct the basis of experimental research and clinical research, deepen the reform, should update thinking, update awareness, update observation, in the reform forward, innovation. Innovation, there must be a challenge to the traditional concept, to overcome its shortcomings, to correct its shortcomings so that it become more perfect. Innovation must challenge the status quo and beyond the status quo. Innovation also searches another way to find a new way to overcome cancer.

Why do I come to the 21st century today, the second 10 years to put forward to attack the cancer to launch a total attack? It is no time to wait and it has to propose to launch the total attack. If it is the chance, it should not miss and it has to propose to launch a total attack.

② **It is recognized**

The original hope in modern oncology, the traditional three treatments such as the surgery and radiotherapy, and chemotherapy can overcome cancer, it seems unlikely to rely on traditional therapy in the radiotherapy, chemotherapy to overcome cancer. Why cannot radiotherapy and chemotherapy overcome cancer? It is because its treatment target is only the relief (CR, PR), remission is not cured, but it is just the short-term that is a few weeks of improvement, then it will progress, increase, transfer. How to do? It must be reformed and have the innovation and develop. Can not is it relied on to overcome cancer? should it have another way? Current treatment of the status quo is wandering before, how do? The way out is to reform.

Surgical treatment of traditional therapy is still the main treatment of solid tumors, is the main science and technology of conquering cancer in the future.

(1) _**Recognizing that more than 90% of the cancer is caused by environmental factors or closely related**_ to; in our city, "two-oriented society" construction has a great relevance to the prevention of cancer cancer, cancer control and it is proposed to launch a total attack and to adhere to the road of the prevention of cancer and cancer control with Chinese characteristics "two-styles of the Society.

① building energy-saving emission reduction, environment-friendly "two-oriented society" has a great relevance to the prevention of cancer and controllingcancer

The current province, the city is ongoing energy-saving emission reduction, pollution reduction and building a "two-oriented society" is the governance of environmental pollution, people and social environment are harmony, will greatly reduce the air, water, food contaminants and carcinogenic substances, therefore, the construction of "two-oriented society" has a great relevance to the prevention of cancer and cancer control.

Human beings is in the search for cancer etiology and factors in the process and carried out extensive exploration and accumulated a wealth of knowledge and the most prominent of which it is found that more than 90% of the cancer are caused by environmental factors or closely related.

The United Nations Health Organization: 1/3 of the cancer can be prevented; 1/3 of the cancer can be cured by early treatment; 1/3 of the cancer can be effective treatment to alleviate the symptoms and prolong life. Therefore, it can be considered that cancer can be prevented.

It is important to be aware of the importance of cancer prevention, environmental factors and inappropriate social behavior are important pathogenic factors that may or may not be avoided by these external or human factors.

Through energy-saving emission reduction, pollution prevention, pollution control, construction of "two-oriented society", people improve their health knowledge, environmental pollution and other carcinogenic factors for effective intervention, it will reduce the incidence of cancer.

② adhere to the road of the prevention of cancer and cancer control with the Chinese characteristics "two types of society".

China's energy-saving emission reduction, the province's "two-oriented society", through efforts, will inevitably achieve the great results at the same time to reduce the incidence of cancer. This is the Chinese cancer prevention and cancer control characteristics, is the road of the prevention of cancer and cancer control with Chinese characteristics of "two-oriented society". After 3-5 years of obtaining the experience of successful work in the province and the city from building a "two-oriented society" combined with the path of the prevention of cancer and cancer control of the Chinese characteristics, it can be introduced to the country and the world.

It is a great opportunity to carry out the excellent situation of energy-saving emission reduction, it is a golden opportunity to carry out the prevention of cancer and anti-cancer work; if it is missed, it will no longer come, so I proposed the basic imagination and designs to overcome cancer and launch the attack and it was put forward a comprehensive planning and layout of the basic design of the framework.

(3) **recognize and the building of a well-off society and everyone is healthy away from cancer and the way-out of the prevention of cancer and control cancer lies in prevention; in urbanization and rural areas, it is to adhere to the road of the Chinese characteristics of the prevention and anti-cancer and it is put forward the need for general attack.**

By 2020, we will achieve a grand goal of building a well-off society in an all-round way. The people's living standard has been improved. The construction of resource-saving and environment-friendly society has made great progress. We should build a well-off society in an all-round way. We should adhere to the " Cancer innovation path in rural urbanization anti-cancer work which goes into the community, seize the opportunity to deepen the reform of important areas, so that it is to make "two-oriented society" prevention of cancer and cancer control work go into the community. Everyone is healthy and away from cancer.

2, how to set up the basic idea and design of launching a total attack and conquering cancer

How to overcome the cancer and to launch a total attack? Xu Ze (Professor Xu Ze) proposed the following basic ideas:

(1) how to overcome cancer? It must establish a "cancer animal experimental center"

To overcome cancer → conquer cancer → capture cancer, we must first understand the basic understanding of cancer: the cause of cancer, pathogenesis, pathophysiology, immunopathology, cancer cell biological behavior? Transfer mechanism? Why implant ? Recurrence mechanism? A series of oncology and tumor-related issues have not yet clear. The scientific research of oncology is a virgin land and need to have a lot of basic scientific research and clinical basic research; to carry out basic research in cancer science is the urgent needs of the current oncology.

Therefore, we must establish a "cancer animal experimental center".

To carry out the basic research of oncology, a good laboratory is the key, scientific design, scientific vision, must be through laboratory experiments, in order to draw conclusions, the results.

To transform the research design into scientific research results must have a good laboratory.

We believe that the construction of a scientific base for the construction of a total attack on cancer (science city) must first vigorously build a laboratory so that many basic problems have experimental research, open up the basis of research on oncology and it should encourage the development of new areas of research and product Talent and the result to help capture cancer.

The basic research in medical science is very important to the progress made in the fight against cancer. If there is no breakthrough in basic research, the clinical efficacy is difficult to improve.

The government should open up new areas of research, fight cancer, develop new products, new industries, and realize the new knowledge of these tasks from basic science research.

The current "oncology" is the most backward of the medical disciplines of a discipline, why? Because the "tumor" the name of the disease are not defined, there are various names? Some people write "tumor", "malignant tumor", "new creature", "cancer lumps", "cancer", "cancer" ... ... and so on, to define a disease name, you must understand the cause, pathogenesis, pathology, But the etiology and pathogenesis and pathophysiology of "oncology" are not yet clear and need to have a lot of basic scientific research and clinical basic research. To carry out cancer experimental scientific research is the urgent need of the current oncology discipline.

How can we overcome cancer? How can we start the total attack? A good laboratory is the key. If there is no good laboratory, although there are talent, there are topics, there are projects, there are funds, if not the experiment, it can only be fantasy, empty talk, can not be a result, can not be accomplished.

Experimental surgery in the development of medical science is extremely important, it is to open a closed area of the key medicine, many diseases prevention and control methods are after many times the experimental study, and achieved a stable results before use in clinical and promote the development of medical career.

Why do we have an animal experimental study and establish the Cancer Animal Experimental Center?

The purpose of medical research is to study the disease, to understand the disease, to seek new methods, new technologies, new theories to improve the level of medicine, prevention and treatment of disease. However, the characteristics of medical research is characterized by its research object is the human body itself, and its research results and applied to the human body. Therefore, the results must be strict scientific, accurate and reliable, harmless to the human body. People are the most valuable, many experiments and observations do not allow the researchers in accordance with the wishes of the human body directly to the test, the need to use simulation methods, the establishment of animal models, experimental research. To be fully harmless to the human body after the success of animal experiments on the basis of success, can be applied to clinical, applied to the human body.

In order to overcome the cancer, start the total attack, we must establish a cancer animal experimental center, the laboratory must be related to good equipment, conditions, experimental personnel need to concentrate on, can calm downand carry out experimental research work, we must attach importance to the "three bases and three stricts."

(2) how to overcome cancer? It must be the founder of "innovative molecular cancer medical school", training personnel, training the relevant personnel who can participate in conquer cancer and launch the total attack and talent must be genuine talent.

Personnel must have knowledge of medical college, must also have life science knowledge, genetic engineering, molecular biology, environmental science, environmental science, Chinese medicine knowledge, medical multidisciplinary knowledge, immunology, endocrinology, virology, immunopharmacology … … and so on.

The current tumor hospital or the top three hospital cancer department most have the medical, radiotherapy, chemotherapy, comprehensive … … and other knowledge and the talent status is now mainly radiotherapy, chemotherapy and other professionals.

To overcome the cancer, talent is the key, how to cultivate talent is the key, the study of cancer requires a number of disciplines of knowledge and technology and genetic engineering, molecular biology, virological experimental personnel; to have knowledge must also have technology and it is to have the ability to operate; to have technology needs to have knowledge so that under the guidance of the theory it is to develop the high-end technology and it needs to have the first-class talent of conquering the tackle, we must concentrate on, calm down, concentrate on this work; where is talent from ?it is based on our own training and the own machine hatchs talent.

In order to overcome the cancer, to launch a total attack, the people who future participation or commitment to the work must have the necessary knowledge and technology.

In view of the fact that more than 90% of the cancer is caused by environmental factors or closely related to, in the current we are ongoing resource-saving and environment-friendly society to build a comprehensive test of energy-saving emission reduction, sewage treatment, this policy and work have a great relevance with prevention of cancer and cancer control work, we must cultivate the relevant personnel.

Therefore, we must build innovative molecular cancer medical school and experimental secondary school talent. In the 21st century the modern high-tech knowledge was summarized as three aspects: life science knowledge; environmental science knowledge; information science knowledge.

The current educational content can not keep up with the development of the times. To overcome the total attack of cancer, we must develop modern high-tech disciplines, must have a good laboratory, but in the current it is lack of laboratory talent. In order to prevent cancer and cancer control and to construct the "two-oriented society" and to conquer cancer, it is not the lack of college graduates, graduate students, but the lack of modern high-tech middle-level specialist talents with the laboratory experiments experience who can go deep into the community to carry out the general attack and to prevent cancer and to control cancer.

Therefore, it is proposed that it must be founded:

① founder of "innovative molecular cancer medical school", training modern high-tech senior cancer doctor (four years college).

② "innovative modern high-tech experimental life science and technology college" (secondary three-year system)

Foster the establishment of laboratory personnel for tertiary institutions. Modern life science and technology progresses rapidly, genetic engineering, molecular biology, cell inheritance rapid develop.

③ founder of "modern high-tech environmental science and technology college" (secondary school three years)

Environmental science has attracted the attention of the world, it will be emerging disciplines, new industries, the current energy-saving emission reduction, pollution control, building a "two-oriented society" must conduct a large number of research topics for the research, use modern high-tech talent in-depth community, to develop the work of combined with prevention of cancer and anti-cancer.

(3) how to overcome cancer? It must have the practice base of be implemented to overcome the cancer and launch a total attack, must "build the hospital of the prevention and treatment of cancer during the whole process of development and occurrence of cancer " - global demonstration of cancer prevention and treatment hospital.

Why is the global demonstration of cancer prevention and treatment research? It is because it was the first time in the world that the XZ-C had launched an initiative to attack the cancer, which was presented in his 38th chapter in the edition of the New Concept and New Approach to Cancer Therapy published in 2011.

Professor Xu Ze in March 2013 proposed "the design and feasibility report to build Wuhan anti-cancer prevention and treatment of hospital " - to elaborate the necessity and feasibility of the establishment of the whole hospital,.

(See full text)

(4) how to overcome cancer? We must establish a "Institute of Innovative Molecular Cancer" to carry out multidisciplinary research related to cancer and set up a related specialist group. In order to overcome the cancer, improve the cure rate, reduce the mortality rate, improve the quality of life, improve the medical level, reduce the complications, the basic research must be carried out.

The study of oncology is the most complex and difficult problem in medical research. It involves multidisciplinary knowledge and theory, including pathology, cytology, immunology, virology, endocrinology, medical genetics, immunopharmacology, molecular Oncology; from the molecular level of the tumor pathogenesis to understand the causes of the disease it will be to provide effective intervention and the treatment measures for the prevention and treatment.

In view of the study of oncology involving multidisciplinary knowledge and theory, we must set up the relevant specialist group, further study, based on the knowledge and theory of the discipline, known medicine, to explore the unknown knowledge of the discipline, the future of medicine, edge disciplines, interdisciplinary, in order to help overcome cancer.

It should be set up following the cancer and is closely related to the specialist group, special in-depth basis and clinical research.

① Immunology and Cancer Research Group

The study group of recent clinical research tasks should be: a, the assessment of the immune function of cancer patients; b, the efficacy of immunoregulatory treatment of cancer patients monitoring; c, put, chemotherapy in patients with immune function quantitative measurement.

② Virus and Cancer Research Group

Some of the cancer known to be closely related to the virus, the treatment should be considered the corresponding treatment, and the virus is closely related to human tumors are: Burkitt Muba; nasopharyngeal carcinoma; leukemia; breast cancer; cervical cancer; Gold lymphoma and so on.

The study of the etiology of human tumor has progressed rapidly in recent years. If you can prove that some of the human tumor virus causes, it is possible to use the vaccine to prevent the occurrence of cancer and control its popularity.

③ Endocrine hormone and cancer research group

Hormone is an important chemical substance that regulates the development and function of the body, and the hormones maintain a dynamic equilibrium relationship according to the law of unity of opposites. Endocrine disorders, due to the imbalance of hormones, so that some hormones continue to act on a tissue, this abnormal chronic stimulation may lead to cell proliferation and cancer.

A carcinogenic hormone can only promote the growth of tissue cells, such as ovarian estrogen, pituitary gonadotropin. Experimental studies have shown that hormonal imbalance caused by thyroid, pituitary, ovary, testis, adrenal cortex and the palace, cervix, vagina, breast and other organs of the tumor, estrogen has caused the role of breast cancer.

④ mycotoxin and cancer research group

it is necessary to have a further study on the carcinogenic factors of some known tumors closely related to mycotoxi. In the recent ten years, some mycotoxins are gradually observed to have carcinogenic or cancer-promoting action on animals. Therefore, medical circle begin to pay more and more attention to studying the relation of fungus and its mycotoxin with human tumor.

Mouldy grains polluted by Aflatoxin in a liver cancer-prone area of China are mixed in feed to feed rats. After six moths, the inducing rate of liver cancer is up to 80%. This kind of feed can also cause monkeys' liver cirrhosis as well as other hepatic lesions and induce liver cancer. Most of the induced liver cancers are hepatocellular cancers. Furthermore, this kind of feed can lead to the adenocarcinoma of kidney, stomach and colon; intratracheal instillation can cause squamous cell carcinoma of lung.

Therefore, making a good job of mould proofing and ridding of oil and foodstuffs is important for exploring the prevention of some tumors and ensuring popular physical fitness.

In the esophageal cancer-prone area of China, Geotrichum candidum Link abstracted from edible pickled vegetable is proved to have the cancer-promoting action. Use the culture of Geotrichum candidum Link to feed rats for twenty months, and then papilloma in anterior stomach is induced. Some moldy food can cause precancerous lesion and early cancer in esophageal epithelium of animals

⑤ Environmental and Cancer Research Group

During the process of seeking for the cause of cancer and occurrence conditions, human have carried out an extensive research and accumulated rich knowledge, which have found that above 90% cancers are caused by or closely related to environment.

How to prove the relationship between environmental pollution and cancer? there are many examples of history; air pollution, water pollution, soil pollution, food pollution have the serious impact on human carcinogenesis.

The above study group composed of various schools

(5) **how to overcome the cancer to attack the total attack? It must "set up the medical, teaching, research, science city to overcome the cancer and launch a total attack"**

We strive for "to build Wuhan Science City to attack the cancer and launch a total attack"

The basic Envisage and design of XZ-C's launching the total attack

Xu Ze Professor proposed the following of the general idea of the total attack of conquering cancer and the basic design of science city

<u>Dawn spirit of scientific research</u>

<u>Hard work and struggle</u> ------18 years of cold window, hard work

↓

<u>Review and reflection</u> -------------Follow-up, summed up the successful experience of treatment (In the second monograph there are the typical case); reflection failure treatment lessons (in the first monograph there are cases of failing to prevent from recurrence, failed to stop metastasis)

↓

open up Innovation 48 kinds of good tumor inhibition rate were screened out of 200 kinds of Chinese herbal medicine in the animal experiments ; 11 years of clinical validation of Z-C immunoregulation of traditional Chinese medicine series; it was realized to rise to theoretical knowledge, new concepts, new models.

↓

Facing future medicine ------ Recognizing the inadequacies and problems of traditional therapies in the twentieth century,recognize the direction of the 21st century

↓

Look forward to look ------------ Suggest:

- Establishment of Innovative Molecular Tumor Hospital

- Cultivating advanced cancer researchers for the country.
- Establishment of innovative molecular tumor hospital (at the molecular level of Western medicine combined)
- benefit more cancer patients and serve more cancer patients.
- Establishment of Innovative Molecular Cancer Institute
- Research cells begin to change
- to the CT can be found between a long time,

To achieve three early goals,

"Target" metastasis, cancerous lesions, precancerous state.

- Build innovative molecular cancer pharmaceuticals
- out of a new way to overcome the cancer with our characteristics

Medicine and teaching and research and development science city

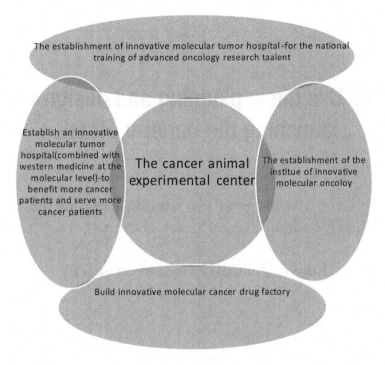

- The establishment of innovative molecular tumor hospital - for the national training of advanced oncology research talent.

- Establish an innovative molecular tumor hospital (combined with Western medicine at the molecular level) - to benefit more cancer patients and serve more cancer patients.

- The establishment of the Institute of Innovative Molecular Oncology - Research on cell initiation of malignancy - to CT can be found between a long period of time to achieve three early goals, "target" metastasis, cancer lesions, precancerous state.

- Build innovative molecular cancer drug factory - out of a new path with cancer of our country.

The mode of the science base of conquering cancer and launching the total attack (The science city)

XZ-C 's basic planning and design of launching the general attack

Professor Xu Ze (XU ZE) proposed the overall design of the Science City to overcome cancer and launch the general attack of cancer

Dawn Scientific research spirit

Hard work

20 years of hard work, hard work

Review and Reflection

1. Follow-up and summary of successful treatment experience (typical cases in the second monograph);

2. Rethinking the lessons of treatment failure (the first monograph failed to prevent recurrence and failed to prevent metastasis).

Open up and Innovation

For 200 kinds of Chinese herbal medicine in Animal experiments, screened 48 species with good tumor inhibition rate. 20 years clinical validation of XZ-C immunomodulation Chinese medicine series preparations, and realized and raised up to theoretical knowledge, new concepts, new models

Future-oriented medicine

Recognizing some of the shortcomings and problems of traditional therapy in the 20th century, Recognize the direction of the 21st century.

Look forward to the future

Suggest:

- Establish an innovative molecular oncology hospital – to train high-level oncology research talents for the country.

- Establish innovative molecular cancer cancer occurrence and development, prevention and treatment of hospitals (in combination with Western medicine at the molecular level) - to benefit more cancer patients and serve more cancer patients.

- The establishment of an innovative molecular tumor research institute - research cells begin to malignant - to CT can be found for a large period of time to achieve the three-early target, "target" metastasis, cancer lesions, precancerous state.

- Establish an innovative molecular tumor drug factory – stepping out of a new path to overcome cancer with Chinese characteristics.

- Establish an environmental protection and cancer prevention research institute and carry out anti-cancer system engineering

(6) The theoretical system of XZ-C immunomodulation and cancer treatment has been formed.

Professor Xu Ze has published self-reliance and hard work for 60 years in the book "New Concepts and New Methods of Cancer Treatment". Nearly 100 scientific research papers on a series of basic and clinical research findings have been published and published in the form of a new book.

This book has formed the theoretical system of XZ-C immune regulation and treatment of cancer, and the clinical basis and experimental basis for cancer treatment are undergoing clinical application observation and verification.

The findings from XZ-C laboratory animal experiments

A. Removal of the thymus can produce cancer-bearing animal models

B. During cancer progression, namely showed progressive atrophy

Find the cause: thymic atrophy, immune dysfunction

Proposed the theoretical basis of treatment:
XZ-C Immune Regulation and Control
Protect Thymus and increase immune functions

Exclusive development of products: XZ-C immunomodulatory agents 1-10

Clinical validation:
30 years, outpatient follow-up and observation for the more than 12,000 cases
In the advanced cancer patients, and the effective of treatment is satisfactory

Theoretical System of XZ-C immune regulate and control of cancer therapy

XZ-C Theoretical System for Immunomodulation and Treatment of Cancer (XZ-C) (XU ZE-China)

XZ-C (XU ZE-China, Xu Ze - China) basic idea and design for launching the general attack

Shuguang scientific research spirit

Hard struggle

——20 years of cold window, hard work

Review and reflect

—— Follow-up, summarizing the successful experience of treatment (a typical case in the second monograph); rethinking the lessons of treatment failure (the first monograph failed to prevent recurrence and failed to prevent metastasis).

Open up and Innovation

—— 200 kinds of Chinese herbal medicine experiments screened out 48 clinical trials with good tumor inhibition rate and Z-C immunomodulation Chinese medicine series preparations, and realized the rise to theoretical knowledge, new concepts and new models.

Future-oriented medicine

—— Recognizing the shortcomings and problems of traditional therapy in the 20th century, recognizing the direction of the 21st century.

Looking forward

—— Recommendations:

- Establish an innovative molecular tumor hospital

- Establish an innovative molecular tumor hospital.

- Established an innovative molecular tumor research institute.

- Establish an innovative molecular tumor drug factory.

- Establish an innovative environmental protection and cancer prevention research institute.

The Scientific base to overcome cancer and to launch the general attack of cancer (the Science City)

The scientific base of conquering cancer and launching the general attack to cancer(the scientific city) including :

Innovation molecular tumor hospital

and modern high tech and science talents

Creative and innovation

molecular tumor Chinese

and western combination

hospital

Cancer animal experimental center

Innovation molecular

tumor research institution

Innovation molecular tumor Nami

Preparation pharmaceutics

Medical education research and development science city or science base

At the age of 85, he published the medical monograph "Condense Wisdom and conquer cancer ----for Benefiting Mankind", XZ-C proposed that " How to overcome cancer? How can I prevent cancer? I see; how to treat cancer? By my opinion".

Professor Xu Ze proposed the engineering planning diagram of how to conquer cancer.

This medical monograph is a practical, applied, research-oriented, implementation of how to overcome the outline of cancer. This set of scientific research programs, scientific research design, scientific research planning, and blueprints can be used by countries, provinces, and states to implement the vision of conquering cancer and benefit humanity.

This implementation outline of the main project is:

1. Conquer cancer and launch the total attack ; Put the equal attention to cancer prevention and cancer control and cancer treatment

2. Create a scientific research base for multidisciplinary and cancer-related research – The Science City.

The two-wing project is:

A wing - how to prevent cancer? To reduce the incidence of cancer

B wing - how to treat cancer? To improve cancer cure rate

Aims:

A: Reduce the incidence of cancer

B: Improve cancer cure rate, prolong patient survival and improve quality of life

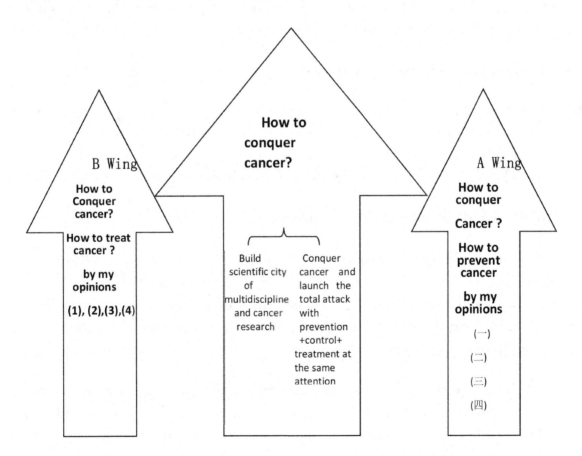

Figure 1. Schematic diagram of XZ-C

How does a country carry out and build a "science city" that overcomes cancer and launches the general attack of cancer?

My initial design and design:

Suggest:

Set up the "National Cancer Working Group"

Each professional working group:

Ministry of Science and Technology

----- Guidance Department of Science and Technology - responsible for the establishment of "Innovative Molecular Oncology Research Institute"

National Ministry of Education

----- Guidance Provincial Department of Education - responsible for the establishment of "Innovative Molecular Oncology Medical School"

National Health and Health Commission

----- Guidance Provincial Health and Health Commission - responsible for the establishment of "innovative molecular level Chinese and Western medicine combined with cancer occurrence, exhibition process prevention and treatment hospital" (cancer full-course prevention and treatment hospital)

The Ministry of Ecology and Environment

------ Guiding the Provincial Department of Ecology and Environment - Responsible for the establishment of the "Environmental Protection and Health Cancer Research Institute", should open up new areas, new technologies and new industries for environmental protection and cancer research *because 90% of cancers occur closely related to the environment.*

It should be from clothing, food, shelter, anti-cancer, from the big environment, small environment to prevent cancer; first, monitor, characterize, quantify, and standardize, establish multi-project laboratories, conduct macroscopic, microscopic, and ultra-microscopic research to study specific methods and measures for preventing cancer.

National Association for Science and Technology

---- Guidance Provincial and Municipal Science Association - Association of Science and Technology Associations, multidisciplinary associations and associations with the Association of Science and Technology, easy to handle multidisciplinary composition of anti-cancer, anti-cancer research groups such as Collaborate with the Society of Viruses to establish a research group on viruses and cancer; Collaborate with the Society for Immunology to establish an immunology and cancer related research group; Can work with the Endocrine Hormone Society;Establish a research group on endocrine hormones and cancer...etc. The school team should establish a laboratory.

In this way, the cancer research teams in various countries will inevitably bloom, the results will be beneficial to the people, benefit the well-off society, everyone's health, and stay away from cancer.

Each province can set up a cancer prevention working group (station), or "province to conquer cancer work office", have full-time staff to work, should be diligent and thrifty, do everything for the people, do good things, do good things for future generations, and seek health and welfare for future generations. In the contemporary, it is beneficial to the future.

六

The necessity and feasibility of in the construction of a well-off society meanwhile it is recommended to build up the "ride scientific research" conducting scientific research of cancer prevention and treatment work for cancer prevention and cancer control

----- Adhere to the anti – cancer and cancer prevention new path of the Chinese characteristics of well-off society

The country is currently implementing the spirit of the 19th Party Congress and ensuring the ambitious goal of building a well-off society nationwide by 2020. The country is building an innovative country and prospering technological innovation.

National Science and Technology Innovation Conference deepens institutional reform and decides to enter the ranks of innovative countries by 2020. Its goal is to achieve a major breakthrough in scientific research in key areas. New achievements in several fields have entered the forefront of the world. The scientific quality of the whole nation has generally improved and entered an innovative country.

This great situation, but also for our capture of cancer for the direction of scientific research work to create a major opportunity to deeply encourage me to actively participate in, pioneering and innovative. I deeply appreciate that cancer should not only pay attention to treatment, but also to pay attention to prevention, in order to stop at the source. The way out of cancer treatment is in the "three early" (early detection, early diagnosis, early treatment), anti-cancer out of the way is in the prevention.

I deeply think that:

In this excellent situation, great opportunity, but also for anti-cancer, anti-cancer research work, creating a good opportunity. Therefore, I suggest: you can engage in "ride research", never missed, when no longer come.

What is "ride car scientific research"?

This is what I thought, and no one in the literature mentioned it. Currently building an ecological civilization and protecting the ecological environment and building a well-off society and building an innovative country are the historic great initiative; It is achievement in the contemporary, and it is beneficial in the future and seeking health and welfare for hundreds of millions of people and a great pioneering work for the health and welfare of future generations. I want to apply for a "scientific research and free ride" under the wheel of great history and bring up research work on cancer prevention and anti-cancer and conquer cancer and it will definitely receive fruitful results and strive to achieve new achievements in the basic and clinical research of cancer treatment in China, and enter the forefront of the world and strive to achieve a major breakthrough in scientific research in the key area of cancer.

In the current energy-saving emission reduction, pollution prevention, pollution control of the excellent situation, is conducive to carry out anti-cancer, cancer control of scientific research and prevention and control work. Environmental and cancer a great relationship, energy saving, pollution abatement, building an environment-friendly society and the prevention of environmental carcinogenesis is closely related. As early as the 20th century, 80 years of domestic and foreign experts, scholars believe that more than 90% of the cancer is caused by environmental factors, protection and recovery of a good environment, is an important part of the prevention of cancer.

I have been engaged in the experimental study of tumor surgery and clinical practice has been half a century. Knowing to achieve the purpose of cancer prevention and control, must be government-led, experts, scholars efforts, the masses to participate, mobilization of the whole people, thousands of households to participate in order to do. At present, China is building an innovative country, building a well-off society, it is the government-led, the masses involved, mobilization of the whole people, thousands of households involved in the work, will be able to improve people's awareness of cancer, to prevent cancer, Our province, the city significantly reduced the incidence of cancer effect.

I would like to suggest:

In the building of a moderately prosperous society, rural urbanization work, the development of prevention of cancer and anti-cancer outline, the development of prevention of cancer and anti-cancer measures, the development of new towns, new rural cancer prevention and control planning and measures. Carry out prevention of cancer and cancer control work. Adhere to the Chinese characteristics of prevention of cancer and cancer control innovation path, to overcome cancer, to built a well-off society and everyone is healthy and staying away from cancer.

Therefore, I would like to put forward a proposal for "ride scientific research":

Building a well-off society, building an ecological civilization and protecting the ecological environment, building an innovative country. This achievement work is in the modern age and benefiting in the future and a historic great initiative for the health and welfare of hundreds of millions of people, take the opportunity to "ride the car research", conduct research and cancer control measures for cancer control and prevention. The purpose is to make people's health, stay away from cancer, and reduce the incidence of cancer in China, our province and our city.

1. **Building a well-off society is conducive to scientific research on cancer prevention and cancer control and its prevention and control work.**

In order to build a well-off society, the construction of new socialist countryside, new towns should also carry out prevention cancer work so that in a well-off society everyone improves prevention of cancer and anti-cancer knowledge, everyone is health and stays away from cancer. In well-off society and the new socialist countryside and the new town how should it be to prevent cancer and anti-cancer? Should it prevent cancer from the clothing, food, shelter or from improving the living environment, or from improving the living habits ? with this basic knowledge, the vast majority of cancer can be avoided and can be prevented.

In order to carry out prevention of cancer and cancer control work, we should first understand and study the relationship between the environment and cancer:

(1) the relationship between environment and cancer

1. air pollution and cancer

Humans have developed tons of tons of coal, oil and natural gas as fuel and energy, such as thermal power generation, smelting steel, automobiles and aircraft, which are producing or discharging and polluting a large amount of harmful gases such as tar, kerosene and dust into the atmosphere surroundings around the clock. Air pollution can cause many diseases to occur, and the most serious is lung cancer.

2. water pollution and cancer

The pollution of water quality is mainly caused by industrial and agricultural production and urban sewage.

3. Soil pollution, food chain and cancer

Large-scale industrial and agricultural production activities of human beings inject a large amount of industrial waste water residue and pesticide fertilizer into the soil, which is deteriorating soil quality, posing a threat to human health and is also a cause of cancer.

China's industrial development has made great contributions to China's economic development. However, at the same time of industrial development, it also brings environmental pollution problems. Measures must be taken actively to strictly control pollution control.

Building a resource-saving and environment-friendly society in a prominent position in the industrialization and modernization development strategy and implementing to each unit, each family. Building an environment-friendly society is an important action to highlight environmental protection and is a top priority for curbing environmental degradation.

At present, we are conducting a comprehensive supporting experiment for resource-saving and environment-friendly society construction to save energy, reduce emissions, and discharge sewage. This policy and work has a great correlation with cancer prevention and control work because:

1. human beings in the search for cancer etiology and factors in the process, carried out a wide range of exploration, accumulated a wealth of knowledge. The most

prominent among them is the discovery of that more than 90% of the cancers are caused by environmental factors or closely related.

At present, our province and our city are carrying out energy conservation and emission reduction, pollution reduction and pollution control, and environmental pollution control. It will greatly reduce pollutants and carcinogens in air, water and food. Therefore, it has a great correlation with prevention of cancer and cancer control.

2. the United Nations Health Organization proposed:

1/3 of the cancer can be prevented; 1/3 of cancer can be cured by early treatment; 1/3 of cancer can be effective treatment and reduce symptoms and prolong life. Therefore, it can be considered that cancer can be prevented.

The importance of cancer prevention must be fully recognized, and environmental factors and inappropriate social behavior are the factors that cause attention.These external or artificial factors can be avoided or interfered with.

Through energy conservation, pollution prevention, pollution control, people have improved their health knowledge and conducted effective interventions for carcinogenic factors such as environmental pollution. It will definitely reduce the incidence of related cancers.

3. Environmental pollution can increase the incidence of cancer:

I deeply understand:

Why are energy-saving and emission-reduction and environmentally friendly "two-type society" engaged in? Because with the development of modern industrialization, a lot of energy consumption, a lot of production, during the course of life, a large amount of harmful gases such as tar, soot, and dust are discharged into the atmosphere around the clock. Atmospheric pollution, water pollution, soil pollution, food pollution, and occupational carcinogens have soared.In recent decades, the incidence and mortality of lung cancer in Western developed countries has increased rapidly. Such as the British lung cancer mortality in 1930 to 100 million, up to 1975 up to 120.3 / 10 million, 45 years, an increase of 12 times. The United States 1934 - 1974 male lung cancer mortality increased from 3.0 / 10 million to 54.5 / 10 million, an increase of 17 times. The above data is amazing. If not energy-saving emission reduction, it will be a lot of emissions of pollutants, greatly harming human health, to promote cancer incidence and mortality rate of rapid growth. Energy-saving emission reduction is for the healthy development of industrialization, continue to leap.

Because environmental pollution is harmful to society and harmful to human life, improving the environment, preventing pollution, and safeguarding health will help build a healthy, happy, harmonious and environment-friendly society. So, what is the danger of environmental pollution? What makes people fear is that environmental pollutants contain many carcinogens, which promotes the rise of cancer incidence.

For example, the damage of nuclear power plants in Japan has led to a significant increase in the concentration of nuclear radioactive materials in the surrounding air, water, soil, and food, which has led to an increase in the incidence of leukemia and cancer, which not only jeopardizes contemporary but also jeopardizes future generations..

4. the harm of environmental pollution:

As we all know, the harm of environmental pollution is:

1). Damage people's health

Radiation, nuclear radiation, bacteria, viruses, harmful chemical poisons, air pollution, water pollution, soil pollution, food pollution, not only damage people's lives, but also lead to an increasing incidence of human cancer;

2). Causing epidemic spread of infectious diseases;

3). A large number of polluting chemicals, harmful gases, harmful water sources, fertilizers, and pesticides can cause cancer and mutation, causing high risk of cancer and high incidence.

Therefore, to reduce the incidence of cancer, we must improve the environment, prevent and control pollution, and build an environment-friendly society and a harmonious society.

The anti-cancer strategy should be prevention of cancer and cancer control, using Class I prevention, Class II prevention, and Class III prevention. I deeply believe **_that the current prevention of pollution and pollution control is a level I prevention_**, and it is a fundamental anti-cancer measure. In fact, under the leadership of the government, the masses have mobilized the mass cancer prevention measures or all the people mobilized to participate in the masses of prevention of cancer measures.

2. It is suggested that while creating a well-off society, we will engage in a "riding car with the scientific research" – conducting medical research of cancer prevention and treatment and cancer prevention and cancer control work.

1). I believe that current energy conservation and emission reduction and pollution prevention and pollution control, which it is a Class I prevention against cancer and cancer control. Its purpose and effect can achieve the level I prevention of cancer. This is a golden opportunity. It is imperative to seize this great opportunity that is once in a lifetime. Time is no longer coming. I have been engaged in experimental basic research and clinical medical practice in oncology surgery for half a century and deeply aware of the purpose of achieving cancer prevention and control cancer, it must be led by the government, the efforts of experts and scholars, the participation of the masses, the mobilization of the whole people, and the work of thousands of households. It will definitely improve the awareness of cancer prevention among the people, achieve the effect of preventing cancer and cancer, and receive the effect of reducing the incidence of cancer in our province and the city.

2). Carrying out prevention of cancer and cancer control, there is currently no practical way. We must not only proceed from the technical and tactical aspects, but must focus on the strategy and implement the people-oriented principle, and fundamentally emphasize the harmony between people and the environment. Scientific research must be carried out to explore and innovate. <u>Science is an endless frontier, and scientific research is endless</u>. With a developmental vision, look forward, under the guidance of the scientific concept of development, carry out scientific research on energy conservation, pollution prevention, treatment and prevention of cancer, cancer control, and reduction of cancer incidence. There will be a lot of new knowledge that is not yet known, even the original innovative research results and the creation of new disciplines and new industries.

I deeply understand this policy and work:

Energy conservation, pollution prevention, pollution control, and pollution control itself essentially contain the significance and effect of preventing cancer and controlling cancer. However, it is not really pointed out. ***I want to make a suggestion, which It is suggested that the province and the city clearly point out that while building a well-off society, it conducts research on cancer control and prevention and develops cancer control plans and measures and raising people's awareness of cancer prevention is also an innovation, and it is also a pioneering work for the benefit of the country and the people.***

To raise people's awareness of cancer prevention, we must have a purpose to build a well-off society. This is the vital interest in caring for the health of the people. It will surely be supported and grateful by the people of the province, and will be more serious and active in energy conservation and emission reduction and prevent pollution work and control pollution work and prevent cancer work and cancer control work.

Prevention of cancer and anti-cancer work are a tough hard bone, but it should continue to linger. Because cancer is a major hazard to humans, prevention of cancer and anti-cancer are human causes. I know that if I want to do this work well, it is impossible to rely on the personal efforts of experts and scholars. It must be mobilized by the government, mobilized by the whole people, and can only be done, and only socialism can do it. It is necessary to get out of the road of anti-cancer and anti-cancer innovation with Chinese characteristics. I am convinced that while building a well-off society, "ride-taking research" will carry out the prevention and control plans for prevention of cancer and anti-cancer prevention and measures of prevention of cancer for group prevention and group control. The cancer incidence and mortality rate of our province and my Wuhan city circle (8+1) will definitely drop significantly.

3. **Follow the scientific development concept and adhere to the innovative road of anti-cancer and anti-metastasis with Chinese characteristics**

Why do I propose that *while building a well-off society, it does a "catch-up or ride scientific research"? Why do you think this is a good time to help "overcome cancer"?*

This is that I gradually recognized from the research work engaged in cancer research during 28 years of research journey. It is our journey of scientific research to complete the application of the "Eighth Five-Year Plan". It is a series of coherent scientific research steps, scientific research stages, scientific research exhibitions, continuous integration, step by step, and different understandings at different stages.

Scientific research climbing is like climbing mountains. When you reach a mountain peak, you can see a layer of scenery. A mountain is taller than a mountain. A mountain is better than a mountain.

Following the scientific development concept, the ideological understanding and scientific thinking of my scientific research journey can be divided into three stages briefly introduced as the following:

1, the first stage (1985 - 1999)

New discoveries and new insights – discovering problems – asking questions – innovative thinking and changing ideas.

In 1985, I made a petition to more than 3,000 patients who had undergone chest and abdominal cancer surgery. It was found that most patients relapsed or metastasized 2-3 years after surgery. Postoperative recurrence and metastasis are the key factors affecting the long-term efficacy of surgery. Clinical basic research to prevent cancer recurrence and metastasis must be carried out. Without breakthroughs in basic research, clinical efficacy is difficult to improve. *Since experimental surgery is a key to opening the medical exclusion zone, we established a tumor animal laboratory, set up an experimental surgical laboratory, and conducted a series of experimental tumor research*:

Carry out cancer cell transplantation, *establish a cancer animal model, explore the mechanism and law of cancer invasion, metastasis and recurrence, and find effective measures to regulate cancer invasion, recurrence and metastasis.*

The new discovery

From experimental tumor research it was found:

1. Excision of the thymus can produce a cancer-bearing animal model, the conclusion of the study:

The occurrence and development of cancer has a positive relationship with the thymus of the host.

2. When we studied the relationship between cancer metastasis and immunity in our laboratory, *the experimental results suggest that metastasis is related to immunity.*

3. Experimental studies have found that *as the cancer progresses, the host's thymus is progressively atrophied.*

For further research, based on the experimental surgical laboratory, the Institute of Experimental Surgery of Hubei College of Traditional Chinese Medicine was established in March 1991. Professor Xu Ze is the director and Academician Fu Fazu is a consultant. ***The goals and tasks of its research are taking "Conquer cancer" as the main direction of attack.***

In 1994, we established a special department for oncology clinics. Through the review of clinical medical practice cases and the analysis, evaluation and reflection of postoperative adjuvant chemotherapy, it was found problems:

1 Some patients with postoperative adjuvant chemotherapy failed to prevent recurrence; ① some patients after adjuvant chemotherapy failed to prevent recurrence;

2 Some patients did not prevent metastasis after adjuvant chemotherapy; ② some Patients with adjuvant chemotherapy failed to prevent the metastasis;

3 Some patients have chemotherapy to promote immune failure; ③ some patients with chemotherapy have promoted immune failure.

From the clinical practice case analysis, reflection, why the patient after surgery failed to prevent recurrence and metastasis? From the chemotherapy drug in the cancer cell cycle to analyze and toreflect, from the analysis and the reflection of the chemical drugs to suppress the immune, from the chemical drug resistance to analyze, reflect, it was found that there are problems:

1). In the current chemotherapy there are still some important errors;

2). The current chemotherapy still exists Several major contradictions and it needs to be further studied and improved.

From the follow-up results it was found that postoperative recurrence and metastasis is the key to long-term efficacy of surgery. So we also raised an important question:

clinicians must pay attention to and study of postoperative recurrence, metastasis prevention and control measures to improve postoperative long-term efficacy.

From 1985 to 1999, We conducted a series of experimental and clinical research, review, analysis, and reflection on cancer, and summarized the positive and negative experiences and lessons of success and failure so that the above experimental research and clinical practice review, reflection, analysis of scientific research materials, summary, collection was organized and was published into the first monograph "New Understanding and New Model of Cancer Treatment", published by Hubei Science and Technology Press in January 2001, issued by Xinhua Bookstore Inc.

2. The second stage (after 2001)

Targeting the goals of research and the "target" of cancer treatment is anti-metastasis and it was pointed out that the key to cancer treatment is anti-metastasis.

After 2001, Our research work did the In-depth analysis of what the key to recurrence and metastasis after surgery is ?

Looking back from the 1970s, in view of the recurrence of cancer after surgery the transfer rate is still very high and in order to prevent postoperative recurrence and metastasis, a series of adjuvant chemotherapy is used; even chemotherapy has started before surgery, but the results are not satisfactory. Recurrence and metastasis still occur soon after surgery. Or the patient had the metastasis while doing chemotherapy ; the more the chemotherapy and the more metastasis. Some cases promotes immune failure due to intensive chemotherapy.

These are all worthy of our clinicians to think and analyze objectively and objectively. How should cancer treatment work prevent recurrence and metastasis to achieve good long-term treatment? Which or which part is blocked or hit will achieve the goal or the purpose of anti-metastasis?

We spent more than three years experimenting with animal models of cancer metastasis, observing and tracking the regularity of cancer cells on the way to metastasis, looking for ways to interfere with and prevent cancer cells from metastasizing. Through the review, analysis and evaluation of a large number of cases in clinical practice, it was proposed:

1   The key to current cancer research is anti-metastasis;

2   Cancer appears in three forms in the human body, and this third form is cancer cells on the way to metastasis;

3   The goal of cancer treatment should be targeted to these three forms;

4   "Two-point, one-line theory" cancer treatment in the whole process of cancer development, not only should pay attention to two points, but should also pay attention to cutting off the front line;

5   The specific measures to prevent metastasis should be to carry out the surrounding, chasing, blocking and intercepting of cancer cells during the metastasis; *put forward that the third field of anticancer metastasis treatment and the main battlefield of cancer cells on the way to metastasis is in the blood circulation and it is important to improve immune regulation and immune surveillance*.

Until 2005, we have compiled a large amount of information on the above experimental research and clinical acceptance and summed up, collected and published the second monograph "New Concepts and New Methods for Cancer Metastasis Treatment" and it was published in January 2006 by the People's Military Medical Press, issued by Xinhua Bookstore; in April 2007, he was awarded the "Three One Hundred" Original Book Awards by the General Administration of Press of the People's Republic of China.

3. The third stage (after 2006)

The research focuses on the prevention and treatment of the whole process of cancer occurrence and development. Closely combined with clinical practice, it aims at the problems and drawbacks of current clinical traditional therapy, and proposes reform and innovation, research and development. Recognizing that the strategy of cancer prevention and treatment must move forward, *the way out for cancer treatment is "three early", and the way out to fight cancer is prevention*.

The second monograph had been moving forward based on the first monograph of scientific research. Targeting the "target" of cancer treatment is to anti-metastasis. *It is pointed out that the key to cancer treatment is anti-metastasis. It is quite correct.*

But the metastasis is just the final late stage during the whole process of the cancer occurrence and development and it is only a partial problem in the whole process of cancer occurrence and tt does not reduce the incidence of cancer occurrence and may reduce mortality.

After 2006, we realized that the goal of cancer treatment is all necessary for the treatment of severely ill patients in the middle and late stages, but the curative effect is very poor. The more new patients are treated, the more the patients show up. Once diagnosed, it is in the middle and late stage, and the effect is not good.

In order to overcome cancer, it must be "three early" and must be prevented in order to reduce the incidence of cancer and cancer mortality.

The way out for cancer treatment is "three early", and **the study of** "three early" must be strengthened.

The occurrence and development of cancer experience the stage of susceptibility - precancerous lesions - the invasive stage; at present, the treatment of cancer in oncology or tumor centers in various cancer hospitals or major hospitals in China, are mainly in the middle and late stages, and the treatment effect is poor. If the middle and late stage patients can operate, they will be treated surgically. If surgery is not possible, only it is used the estimating or conserving the treatment. Therefore, the way out for cancer treatment should be "three early"------Early detection, early diagnosis, early treatment. Early patients generally have better therapeutic effects and improved treatment results. It will inevitably reduce the cancer mortality rate.

Therefore, we must pay attention to the study of early diagnosis methods and treatment methods, but also must pay attention to the treatment of precancerous lesions to reduce the middle and late stage patients in the invasion stage.

If we can treat well in precancerous lesions or early stage cancer, the number of patients who progress to invasion and metastasis will decrease, which will also reduce the incidence of cancer.

Therefore, we believe that the current cancer hospitals or oncology departments, mainly treat patients in the middle and late stages, even if the treatment results are good, it can only reduce the mortality rate and ignore the pre-cancerous lesions in the susceptible stage and early patients, it is impossible to reduce the incidence of cancer.

Therefore, we believe that we must pay attention to the prevention and treatment of cancer occurrence and development during the whole process, which is a strategic global concept. We must update our thinking and change our mindset.

I have been engaged in oncology surgery for 62 years, and the number of patients is increasing. The incidence of cancer is also rising, which makes me deeply understand that cancer must not only pay attention to treatment, but also pay attention to prevention, in order to stop at the source.

*__Therefore, I deeply understand that the cancer treatment is in the "three mornings". Research on "three early" (early detection, early diagnosis, early treatment) must be strengthened. The way to fight cancer is prevention.__*Research on preventive measures must be strengthened.

As mentioned above, the focus of the cancer prevention and treatment strategy is shifted forward. __Its meaning has two aspects, one is to change the way of life and improve prevention measures such as environmental pollution; the other is to treat precancerous lesions and prevent their progression to the invading or mid-late stages__.

The way to control cancer lies in prevention, and research on preventive measures must be strengthened.

Cancer has become a major public health problem worldwide, and cancer prevention and control will face greater challenges than other chronic diseases.

In the past 30 years, China's cancer mortality rate has risen sharply and has become the leading cause of death for urban and rural residents. On average, one in every four deaths has died of cancer.

Cancer is not only a serious threat to human health, but also an important factor in the rise in medical costs. China's annual direct cost for cancer treatment is nearly 100 billion yuan. The patient and the society as a whole bear a huge economic burden. Many patients have spent tens of thousands or even hundreds of thousands of dollars, and they have not achieved corresponding effects. Cancer mortality remains for the first place, what should I do? It is worthy of our clinician analysis, reflection, and research. How is the road to research go? Be sure to recognize the problems that exist in current treatments.

Although countries have invested heavily in the treatment of cancer patients, the 5-year survival rate of some common cancers has not improved significantly in the past 20 years.

How to do? The way to control cancer lies in prevention, prevention and intervention are the top priority in the field of public health.

In recent years, it has been recognized that <u>more than 90% of cancers</u> are caused by environmental factors, and protecting and restoring a good environment is an important part of preventing cancer. One third of cancers are preventable.

The relationship between environment and cancer is extremely close. Environmental pollution can cause various carcinogens to enter the human body or various carcinogenic factors affect the human body. *<u>How to prove the relationship between environmental pollution and cancer has been confirmed by many examples in history.</u>*

<u>Air pollution</u> in environmental pollution can increase the incidence of lung cancer. In industrialized countries, harmful gases such as power generation, steelmaking, automobiles, aircraft, fuel, energy, and large amounts of smoke are emitted into the atmosphere, polluting the air, leading to an increase in the incidence and mortality of lung cancer.

<u>Water</u> pollution and cancer in environmental pollution, water pollution is mainly caused by industrial and agricultural production and urban sewage. Water pollution can induce or promote cancer.

<u>Chemical carcinogenesis</u> in environmental pollution is also closely related to the incidence of cancer. 80-90% of human cancers are related to environmental factors, mainly chemical factors.

Studying the sources of environmentally-contaminated carcinogens and studying how to eliminate such pollution is a very important issue in preventing cancer. Prevention of cancer must be prevention of pollution and pollution control.

I believe that energy conservation, pollution prevention and pollution prevention are the first-level prevention of cancer, and the prevention of cancer is at the source. And think this is a good time to help "overcome cancer". I am convinced that building a well-off society will surely achieve the effects of preventing cancer and cancer, and achieving good results, so that the people can be healthy and stay away from cancer.

In order to overcome cancer and conduct cancer prevention and cancer control research, it is necessary to carry out basic and clinical research on anti-cancer metastasis and recurrence, and carry out joint research on multidisciplinary cooperation. It is necessary to establish Wuhan Anticancer Research Association.

With the strong support of the academicians of the ancestors, Xu Ze, Li Huizhen and other professors applied for preparation, after approval by the higher authorities of Wuhan, on June 21, 2009, the Wuhan Anticancer Research Association was established, and then a committee for cancer metastasis and recurrence treatment was established. It established an academic research team for cancer metastasis, academic research, academic research, academic propaganda, academic workshops or academic seminars, and trained a group of senior talents in the province and the city to fight cancer metastasis and treatment.

With the strong support of the academicians Qiu Fazu, Xu Ze, Li Huizhen and other professors applied for preparation, after approval by the higher authorities of Wuhan. On June 21, 2009, the Wuhan Anticancer Research Association was established, and then a committee for cancer metastasis and recurrence treatment was established. Established an academic research team for cancer metastasis, academic research, academic research, academic propaganda, academic workshops or academic seminars, and trained a group of senior talents in the province and the city to fight cancer metastasis and treatment.

The goal of cancer control research:

The foothold is "research". Under the guidance of the scientific development concept, with a developmental vision and the spirit of innovation, Looking forward, facing the future and developing medicine, it is to study prevention of cancer and cancer control, and to study the mechanism of occurrence and development and metastasis and recurrence and prevention and treatment for cancer.

The research route is to find the problem → ask the question → study the problem → solve the problem or explain the problem in order to help overcome cancer.

Our Wuhan Anticancer Research Association and the 8+1 hospitals in Wuhan City Circle formed the 8+1 Anticancer Alliance in Wuhan City Circle, conduct academic seminars and academic exchanges on cancer prevention and cancer control.

The Wuhan Anticancer Research Society visited the Sterling Cancer Institute in Houston, USA in December 2009 for academic exchanges and presented the second monograph "New Concepts and New Methods for Cancer Metastasis Treatment" and " altas or Analysis of Cancer Metastasis Experiments".

By 2010, we compiled a large amount of research and clinical data from the above experiments and clinical studies, summarized, compiled and published the third monograph "New Concepts and New Methods for Cancer Treatment", published in October 2011 by the People's Military Medical Press and published by Xinhua Bookstore.

The third monograph, "New Concepts and New Methods for Cancer Treatment," is a new concept and innovation. It has both experimental research and clinically validated "new concepts of cancer treatment ", which came up with a series of cancer treatment reform and innovation.

4. Adhere to take the Chinese characteristics of building a well-off society, and at the same time carry out the innovation road of prevention of cancer and cancer control

Through hard work, China's energy conservation and emission reduction, pollution prevention and pollution control, building a well-off society will inevitably achieve great results in reducing the incidence of cancer. This is the characteristic of prevention of cancer and cancer control in socialist countries. This is an innovative way of building a well-off society with Chinese characteristics to prevent cancer and control cancer. After 3-5 years of successful work experience, we can combine the prevention and control and cancer control of our province and our city to build a well-off society. This road of prevention of cancer and cancer-control innovation with Chinese characteristics is pushed to the whole country and pushed to the world.

Why is cancer prevention and cancer control mentioned here? Because more than 90% of cancers are related to environmental pollution and if environmental pollution has improved or changed, it may have the effect of preventing cancer from occurring and controlling the occurrence of cancer. If pollution is controlled, it may prevent or control carcinogens from entering the body.

Both the improvement of the environment and the improvement of the small environment can reduce, prevent or control the effects of environmental carcinogens entering the human body or environmental carcinogens on the human body.

At present, it is a great situation to carry out energy conservation and emission reduction. It is also a great opportunity to carry out research on prevention of cancer and cancer control by "taking a ride on scientific research". It is a great opportunity for a rare event.

In the past, I also realized that prevention of cancer is important, but I can only talk about it on paper and make publicity. Now, under the concrete practice of building a well-off society, anti-cancer and cancer control can be a great time. It can be specifically achieved to reduce the incidence of cancer in our province and the city year by year. It is everyone's responsibility to prevent cancer and control cancer. Medical workers should recognize the burden of their shoulders. Under this great situation, we will do a good job in preventing cancer, improve people's awareness of cancer prevention, change some living habits, and improve some living conditions, and it has environmentally friendly and harmonious life. People will be healthy, happy, long-lived and away from cancer.

In order to do this work well, we created the Wuhan Anticancer Research Association and established a professional committee for anti-cancer metastasis and recurrence and organized more experts, scholars and people with lofty ideals to conduct medical scientific research on cancer prevention and control. I will do my utmost to open up the work of benefiting the country and the people.

Therefore, while doing a good job in energy conservation and emission reduction, pollution prevention and pollution control, and building a well-off society, I make the following suggestions:

Conducting "hitch research", conducting research on cancer prevention and control, and formulating cancer planning and measures (see Annex 2); improve environmental pollution, eliminate or avoid some environmental carcinogenic risk factors, strengthen publicity education on cancer prevention, and popularize cancer prevention knowledge; establish a sound monitoring system to monitor high-risk groups.The government is leading, experts and scholars are working hard, the whole people participate, and the whole people improve their awareness of cancer prevention.

I am convinced that the great results of environmentally friendly and reducing the incidence of cancer in the Wuhan metropolitan area will be achieved.

Energy saving and emission reduction

Pollution prevention and control

Well-off society, away from cancer

Prevention of cancer and control cancer,

conquer cancer

Power and work in the contemporary

Benefits in the future

How to build a well-off society? How to carry out specific measures, guidelines, policies, steps and programs to overcome cancer in building a well-off society?

Government guidance is the key.

Executive talent development is also the key.

Talent must have modern life science knowledge;

There must be modern scientific knowledge and technology for the prevention and treatment of cancer occurrence and development;

It must have prevention cancer and anti-cancer knowledge and technology;

It must also have environmental science knowledge and technology. At present, universities have environmental colleges and life sciences colleges. However, we need modern high-tech high-level and high-level talents with life science knowledge and skills, environmental science knowledge and skills to make the well-off society prevention of cancer, anti-cancer, prevention of pollution, pollution control, scientific and technological innovation experimental research into the colleges and universities laboratory . The experimental talents with strong hands-on ability have enabled the establishment of laboratories in universities and colleges in China.

Therefore, in order to build a well-off society and at the same time "ride scientific research car" to overcome cancer, the cultivation of modern high-tech talent is the key. These modern high-tech intermediate colleges must be established. Wuhan Anti-Cancer Research Association will apply for a modern high-tech life science intermediate college and a modern high-tech environmental science junior college and prepare talents for building a well-off society and conquering cancer and for the scientific innovation, the establishment of high-tech laboratories to train high-tech experimental talents.

I deeply understand that while building a well-off society, we will engage in a "ride-taking research" to build a well-off society and prevent cancer and cancer. It may be a new breakthrough in building a well-off society, and it will also add new content for innovating Wuhan, innovating Hubei, and innovating China for the construction of a national central city.

Several suggestions of building an innovative country to train talents for science and technology innovation and the laboratory construction and the transformation of results

1. Building an innovative country should prosper technological innovation

National Science and Technology Innovation Conference deepened the reform of science and technology system and decided to enter the ranks of innovative countries by 2020. Its goal is to achieve original breakthroughs in key areas of scientific research; Strategic high-tech areas achieve leapfrog development; Innovation achievements in a number of fields have entered the forefront of the world; the scientific quality of the whole nation has generally improved and entered the ranks of innovative countries.

How to build an innovative country? Innovative countries should not only prosper independent innovation, but also prosper original innovation. It should not only catch up with the international advanced level, but also should be at the international leading level.

What is independent innovation?

Independent innovation is a product that people have, we must have it, not rely on others to design and it is our own design and production. Independent innovation is better than others, and superiority is competitive.

What is original innovation?

Original innovation is something that no one else has, or what is not in the world. It is my unique invention, not to learn from others, but to come to us to learn.

Innovation is not only product innovation, but basic theory innovation, and theoretical innovation is a big achievement. Scientific development is based on the innovation of basic theory. This is the big invention and creation, discovering new theories and new laws. For example: Einstein's theory of relativity, Newton's law.

To build a technologically innovative country, we must prosper the fruits of technological innovation and it is not only the results of independent innovation, but also the results of original innovation.

How can we have the results of the scientific and technological innovations?

Talent is the key.

The standard of talent must be true and talented, and both ability and moral integrity.

Whether it is true talent or not must have the result of scientific research and scientific and technological innovation.

How can we have innovative results?

Construction of Laboratory of the corresponding equipment is the key,

With a good laboratory, there are basic conditions for research. Through experimental research, innovative results can be achieved.

How can we have innovative results?

Cultivating talent is not the ultimate goal.

Building a laboratory is not the end goal.

The ultimate goal is to achieve innovative scientific research results and scientific research achievements. The ultimate goal of all research is to achieve scientific research results.

Take or count the heor by the achievement

Take or count the contribution by the achievement

Take or count the academic level

There is the original innovation, it is beyond the international level.

The original innovations must be verified by the new agency.

How can it have technology innovation?

First of all, we must cultivate scientific thinking and scientific thinking.

Have an academic ethos, ask more questions about why? <u>Search the root and Find the reasons, First of all, submit questions, research problem, then solve the problem. Think more about why? Ask more why? Ask how to do? How to perform it? What does it do? To have a scientific and innovative atmosphere, we should cultivate from adolescents.</u>

Teachers at all levels must have scientific thinking and academic ethos and then can train students to ask why? Think more about the problem, analyze the problem. The teacher is the engineer of the human soul; to improve the quality of teaching, we must first improve the level and quality of the teaching staff. First of all, we must improve the academic atmosphere of the teaching staff, scientific and technological innovation thinking and academic level. If the teacher does not have enough knowledge, he will not dare to ask the students why.

2. How can it have technology innovation? Talent is the key.

Where do talents come from and how to cultivate talents?

1. Send people abord to study and after studying outside and returning the country(international students, visiting scholars), participation in scientific and technological innovation and the study of sending countries should dedicate the task of bringing back scientific and technological knowledge. After returning to China, you should produce results and talents.

2. Hiring for coming in. Recruit top-notch scientific and technological talents at home and abroad to host scientific and technological innovation. How to use its talents? How to apply?

1) There should be a better laboratory to enable a group of people to produce scientific and technological innovations.

2) it should be used to train talents, and cultivate a batch of China's own scientific and technological talents, because please come in, will still go, it should be used

for talent incubation, help China to train scientific and technological talents. Even if it comes out of talent, it will produce results.

3) Self-reliance and self-cultivation. If we want to produce original innovations in science and technology, we must cultivate our own scientific and technological talents.

Now that China is the second largest economy in the world, how to continue to develop, how to continue to move forward, leapfrog development, and catch up with the world's largest economy, must be self-reliant and cultivate talents.

To develop modern high technology, we should encourage the development of new research fields, and we must not always run behind others. When people run inside, I run the outer ring:

When people run the outer circle, I will run in the middle circle to surpass the first. Otherwise, running the same circle, people running in front, blocking, you will have difficulty surpassing to the front. So we can't run along the same circle in the same circle (I chose to study the subject always).

Therefore, we must catch up with the world's largest economy. Talent cultivation cannot rely on foreign students studying abroad and visiting scholars to train talents. It is up to China to train talents. We should rely on ourselves to create new technologies, open up new research fields and new industries, and rely on China to train talents.

How to cultivate talents by yourself? First of all, we must cultivate our own talent incubator.

If we want to innovate in science and technology, if we want to leapfrog development, if we want to go to the world's largest economy, it is the key to cultivate innovative talents. If you want to surpass other countries, if you want to open up new research fields, you can't follow other countries' studies. You must rely on your own country to work hard, build ambitions, be ambitious, self-reliant, and cultivate high-level talents for sustainable development.

How to train talents?

The development zone introduces a large number of talents and how to use them to develop their talents. On the one hand, it should be used for technological innovation, development of science and technology, production of results, innovation of products, production, development of new businesses and new industries. On the other hand, the main task is to train talented incubators, train high-tech talents and high-tech leading talents in China, and not only prosper China's scientific and technological innovation, but also make high-tech talents come forth in large numbers.

How to train talents?

I think that a journey of a thousand miles begins with a single step. From now on, we should put our self-reliance and modern high-tech talents on the agenda, and organize self-reliance to train modern high-tech talents. The goal is to surpass the international advanced level and head to the world's first economy. In order to be self-reliant, we must cultivate modern high-tech talents and send them to study abroad, supplemented by visiting scholars (because we could not learn abroad at that time, because China's high technology has already surpassed or kept pace).

Talent training should walk on two legs:

1. One is to attract talents outward. Recruit talents and send personnel to study abroad, visit scholars, and participate in construction and technological innovation after returning to China. Currently, this is an important way to train talents, but this is only a cure, and it can only catch up and it is difficult to surpass.

2. The other is to build a good laboratory on the basis of self-cultivation. In the long run, this is the root cause. You cannot rely on foreign training and you should rely on your own training. In the early days after liberation, China's medical talents were all cultivated on their own. How to cultivate yourself ? it is to set up a laboratory to conduct clinical research and work through animal experiments to reach technological innovation so that we can innovate and surpass .

After the liberation, the medical development of New China, from scratch, is to take this road of self-reliance to cultivate talents and develop jobs.

For example, cardiopulmonary bypass surgery

In the early days after liberation, it was unable to study abroad, visit, communicate or exchange, and there were no foreign medical journals or publications. There are no foreign medical journals and publications. In the late 1950s and early 1960s, several large hospitals in Xi'an, Tianjin, Shanghai, Wuhan, Nanjing, Anyang and other cities jointly formed an extracorporeal circulation open heart surgery animal experiment group. Each group was an animal experiment of cardiopulmonary bypass surgery with hundreds of dogs. After the successful operation of the animal experiment, the Tianjin group also created a half-circulation of extracorporeal circulation. I participated in the Wuhan Animal Experiment Team and organized a delegation to Tianjin, Nanjing, and Anyang to study animal experiments. *China's extracorporeal circulation open heart surgery is based on the animal experiment of the dog to explore the experience of training their own talents.*

Another example is liver transplantation

In the late 1970s, it has not yet established diplomatic relations with the United States and there was not studying abroad, visits, exchanges, and there were no foreign medical journals, publications.

Dr. Dong Fangzhong and Dr. Lin Yanwei in Shanghai Ruijin Hospital and Dr. Qi Fazu and Xia Suisheng in Wuhan Tongji Hospital had established animal laboratories for liver transplantation. At the same time, hundreds of dog liver transplant animal experiments were carried out. All passed the animal experiment and went to the clinic. In Shanghai and Wuhan, both groups of liver transplants have undergone clinical liver transplantation after successful animal experiments. In the 1980s, when the Wuhan Liver Transplantation Results Appraisal Meeting was held, the two groups of animal experiments and clinical trials in Shanghai and Wuhan went hand in hand. Only the Wuhan group is 3 days earlier than the Shanghai group. Clinical liver transplant patients survive for 3 days more. *According to this, the Ministry of Health will focus on liver transplantation in Wuhan and establish an organ transplant research institute.* At that time, I was the drafting leader of the liver transplantation achievement identification expert. I witnessed that the liver transplantation operation in our country also started by cultivating talents through dog animal experiments.

The key to building talents on your own is to build a good laboratory.

The key is that I have a good laboratory. I participated in the extracorporeal circulation animal laboratory in the 1960s. In the 1980s, I established the cirrhosis ascites laboratory.In the early 1990s, I established the Institute of Experimental Surgery to tackle cancer. In my animal laboratory, equipment conditions are good, there are white mice, rats, Dutch pigs, rabbits, dogs, monkeys and other animal experiments, there are better animal sterile operating room which can be used for dog chest, abdomen major surgery and for the animal observation of the hospital after surgery <u>and it can put a variety of designs, ideas, through experimental operations, to achieve results or conclusions</u>

Therefore, the laboratory is a key condition. If no laboratory passes the experiment, it can only be designed and conceived, and it is impossible to be a factual result.

Experimental surgery is extremely important in the development of medicine. It is a key to opening the medical exclusion zone. Many disease prevention methods have been studied in many animal experiments, and the stability results have been applied to the clinic to promote the development of the medical cause.

Therefore, the development of science, technological innovation, and laboratories are key conditions. Self-reliance and self-cultivation of innovative talents, the laboratory is the key condition.

3. How to cultivate talents by yourself?

Talent training mechanism and talent training institution should be established

It should meet the requirements and contents of the modern high-tech talent training mechanism in the 21st century:

1. *<u>Should keep up with the development of modern high technology;</u>*

2. *<u>Keep up with the modern high-tech talents needed in innovative countries and international metropolises.</u>*

Currently we are in the second 10 years of the 21st century and how to recognize and understand the concept and content of modern high technology? Throughout the 20th century, humans have recognized the discovery and application of thermonuclear reactions: the birth and popularity of computers; the establishment and development of molecular biology. It is a major scientific achievement.

The scientific community predicts that leadership science in the 21st century will be a life science with molecular biology as its core; computer-centric information science and environmental science.

Modern high technology will lead new research fields, new industries, and new disciplines. Modern high-tech innovation will lead the future and leapfrog development.

Pedagogy or Education should keep up with the development of the times, and education should be applied. The setting of school specialization should serve the modern high-tech talents needed to build an innovative country and an international metropolis.

Since it is an innovative country, we are striving to be at the forefront of the world, and we must strive for international leading level or international advanced level. Since it is an international metropolis, it must strive to reach the international level, including the level of talent, technology, technological innovation, culture, humanities, knowledge, construction, transportation, etc.

First of all, clear several concepts:

Science and technology refer to science and technology. In a stricter sense, science and technology belong to two different categories. The original meaning of science refers to the theoretical expression of human understanding of the laws of nature, and technology is the means by which mankind transforms the world. *Scientific development has become the main foundation for technological development.*

Generally speaking, the majority of the people use science and technology to understand science, and scientific development and technological progress are linked to people's daily lives through technological achievements.

Characteristics of modern scientific research:

"Theory of science" refers to the science of a basic concept, basic principles and basic laws of comprehensive research, and has a guiding role in applied science, and the development of applied science, in turn, deepens and enriches theoretical science. Sometimes it also refers to general basic science.

*"**Applied Science**"* is a concept that is relative to "theory of science" and refers to science that directly serves production or other social practices. It includes applied theory and applied technology. Applied science is sometimes used as a general term for technical science and engineering science, and it is directly related to the speed of development of the national economy.

*"**Technology" includes two meanings**:*

Various methods of operation developed according to the principles of natural science, such as electrical engineering, welding technology, laser technology, crop cultivation techniques, breeding techniques, and *manufacturing processes or operating procedures.*

In order to build an innovative country, we should prosper scientific and technological innovation. Today we recognize that the development of science and technology and basic research can represent the comprehensive national strength of a country. In other words, it can also represent the comprehensive strength of a national central city.

At present, some provinces and municipal colleges and universities have life science colleges and environmental science colleges. The information science colleges focus on theoretical science, applied science and basic science.

The technical level is mostly in secondary technical schools and secondary vocational schools. In fact, the technical level is very important. Modern high-tech technology is developing rapidly and changing with each passing day. However, at present, China's secondary technical school stays in a single discipline in the 20th century, with outdated equipment and weak teachers, which has not received due attention. The current teaching content cannot keep up with the development of the times. The teaching facilities and teaching content of technical colleges must keep up with the rapid development of modern high-tech technology. Technical colleges are mainly "applied science" and "technology".

Technical science and engineering science, as well as various methods of operation developed according to these scientific principles, as well as the production processes or operating procedures. It is directly related to the speed of development of the national economy.

The level and quality of modern high-tech personnel is also directly related to the sustainable development of China's scientific and technological products. . The level and quality of modern high-tech personnel is also directly related to the sustainable development of China's scientific and technological product quality.

For example, the aerospace industry, the Shenzhou Nine Airlift or God nine and air raises off, the voyage of the sea into the seabed, the high-speed rail… all need modern modern high-tech skills, workers, technicians, engineers; a trace of one minute, one minute and one second must be precise.

In order to build an innovative country to become a science and technology innovation center, we must attach importance to colleges and universities; both ordinary and intermediate science colleges must be equally important. Scientific and technological innovation thinking should be cultivated from young people. Modern high-tech skilled workers and technicians are one of the main players in the development of modern high technology. Therefore, the teaching content and the training of teachers in China's intermediate science colleges must keep up with the development of modern (21st 1920s) high-tech era. For the National Science and Technology Innovation Center, universities, research institutes, and large companies to transport modern high-tech talents and laboratory talents in the 21st century.

Modern high-tech knowledge in the 21st century is summarized in three aspects:

life science and technology knowledge;

environmental science and technology knowledge;

information science and technology knowledge.

The current educational content cannot keep up with the development of the times. In order to develop modern high-tech disciplines, there must be good laboratories, but the current laboratory talents are scarce. The status quo is a lot of doctors and nurse; there are very few people who will catch mice for experimentation. It is not a lack of college graduates, graduate students. It is the lack of modern high-tech intermediate specialists in laboratory experiments. In order to build an innovative country to build a science and technology innovation center, a good laboratory must be built. The construction laboratory must first cultivate laboratory talents. Scientific research talents must be cultivated from young people. *Since ancient times, the hero has been a teenager.*

Therefore, it is recommended to set up a modern high-tech experimental medium-level talent institution in the 21st century to provide talent for building a laboratory.

1. *Established Modern High-Tech Life Science and Technology College (secondary school, three-year system)*

Establishing laboratory talents for colleges and universities.

Modern life science and technology is progressing rapidly, genetic engineering, molecular biology, cytogenetics, and rapid development.

2. *Established a modern high-tech environmental science and technology college (secondary school, three-year system)*

Environmental science has attracted global attention. It will be an emerging discipline, a new industry, the current energy conservation and emission reduction, prevention pollution and pollution control, and the construction of a "two-oriented society". *It is necessary to carry out a large number of scientific research projects, and it is necessary to use modern high-tech technology to carry out prevention pollution and pollution control, ecological balance, food hygiene supervision, etc., and to cultivate a large number of modern high-tech intermediate talents with environmental protection science.*

More than 90% of cancers are caused or closely related to environmental factors. Therefore, the current energy conservation and emission reduction, prevention pollution and pollution control, and the creation of "two-type society" are the first-level preventive measures against cancer and cancer. I hope that I can get the support of the government and train a large number of middle-level professionals in environmental science for the construction of a "two-oriented society."

3. *Founding a modern high-tech information science and technology college (secondary school, three-year system)*

To enrich the construction of laboratories of the respective universities and colleges.

The quality and quantity of information specialists can represent the competitiveness and creativity of a country.

4. How can technology be innovated?

A good laboratory is the key

With talent, it does not mean that there is result or achievement.

With talent, it does not mean that we can prosper technological innovation. Because heroes have the places to use and to apply the skills; scientific research design and scientific research ideas must be performed through laboratory experiment research in order to draw conclusions and to produce the results.

Therefore, scientific and technological innovation must have a good laboratory, the laboratory is the key. If there is no good laboratory, although there are talent personnel, there are topics, there are projects, even if you get hundreds of thousands of dollars, if there is not the experiment, it can only be fantasy, empty talk, cannot have a result.

To turn scientific research design into scientific research results must have a good laboratory.

To compare China's universities with Europe and the United States, the gap between is not the size of the school and the number of teachers and students, the main gap is the lack of high-tech laboratories. Although there are teaching and research groups in all universities in China, namely teaching and research. However, many teaching and research groups have no laboratories, teachers can not conduct experimental research, and they will not be able to produce results and masters.

Science - is the endless frontier, the rapid development of modern high-tech, with each passing day, the quality of university teachers and teaching quality must also keep up with modern high-tech development, advancing with the times.

University teachers should have a dual task on the shoulders, *one is to improve teaching; the second is the development of science.*

University teachers should have a good laboratory for scientific research, follow the scientific concept of development, based on the known science, to explore the unknown science, for the future science, emerging disciplines, border disciplines, interdisciplinary, scientific frontier, innovation, Science hall, brick tiles.

Therefore,

How can China's universities meet international standards?

We should vigorously develop well - established laboratories.

How to fight for our university into the top 500, 200 strong?

We should vigorously develop well - established laboratories.

How to build an innovative country?

It should build a good laboratory.

How can scientific innovation out of the original innovation?

It should build a good laboratory.

How can we open up new research areas?

It should build a good laboratory.

How can basic research be carried out?

It should establish a good laboratory.

How can we fight cancer?

It should establish a good laboratory.

US technology booms, high-tech is developed, the main reason have the more laboratory and the equipment conditions are good; it is paid attention to the science and technology experiments, and attention to the laboratory. China sends a large number of students each year, visiting scholars to the United States to study abroad, graduate students, as visiting scholars, are basically working and studying in the laboratory. The main gap between China University and the United States and Britain and other countries of the University is universities modern high-tech laboratory in the United States and Britain and other with the excellent equipments, teaching and research groups are basically work, research, train graduate students, and guide students in the laboratory so that professors can be innovative results, open up new areas of research, produce a talent and produce a master of science.

At the Massachusetts Institute of Technology, the scale is small, and the number of teachers and students is only a few thousand. However, the school has 38 Nobel Prize winners and won 39 Nobel Prizes in Science.

One of them won the Nobel Prize twice and was r anked the top ranked universities in the world. Because the school has many modern high-tech high-level laboratories, laboratories, and many academic masters, it has developed many cutting-edge research fields, and the study style is strict, strict and rigorous.

This shows that the importance of modern high-tech laboratories in technological innovation;the importance of the laboratory in achieving scientific research results;the importance of laboratories in the development of science.

The laboratory is an incubator for scientific research results; the laboratory is an incubator for talent training.

With a good laboratory, the scientific and technological achievements can be made, and talents can be used by heroes to be talented. Therefore, the base for developing science, prospering technological innovation, and prospering scientific and technological achievements is the laboratory.

There are many colleges and universities in China. There are many teaching and research groups in the subordinate and provincial universities, and a large number of graduate students are also trained. However, some teaching and research groups do not have laboratories or research laboratories. Strictly speaking, it should only be called the teaching group, teaching and not researching. There is no laboratory or research room in the university teaching and research group. How to conduct research? A large number of graduate students have been recruited. How to train and guide graduate students to do experiments and research projects? The teaching and research group does not have a laboratory or research room. The professors can only prepare lessons, lectures, and cannot do experiments or research projects. University professors should not only talk about the known knowledge in textbooks, but also the new developments, new trends in development, new achievements and unknown knowledge. If the teacher does not have a laboratory or research room, he or she cannot conduct research on the subject and obtain scientific research results. I have no place to do experiments, how to guide graduate students to do experiments?

Now a tutor may recruit several graduate students to guide students on how to choose a topic, how to design a project, how to experiment, and how to achieve results or conclusions. However, there are quite a few faculty members who do not have laboratories or research laboratories.

How to guide the experimental operation of graduate students? It is reasonable to say that a tutor should have a good laboratory, it is possible to guide graduate students to conduct scientific research, write papers, and develop science.

In order to develop science and technological innovation, the laboratories are key conditions..

We should vigorously build laboratories, train high-tech talents, and produce more innovative results.

It is therefore recommended that:

1. *subordinate institutions of higher learning should have 1-3 state-level key laboratories*

2. *provincial institutions of higher learning should have 1-3 provincial key laboratories*

3. *municipal institutions of higher learning should have 1-3 municipal key laboratories*

Laboratory rating should be assessed according to the outcomes of level of talents and results

- *National key laboratories should have international leading or international advanced level achievements, and be the leaders of scientific research, and be the masters of science.*

The results must be appraised by the appraisal, and the original results must be verified by the provincial search agency and accepted by the higher authorities.

- *If the international level results cannot be achieved in three years, the level should be lowered and resumed after the corresponding results are obtained.*

- *Provincial key laboratories should have domestically leading or domestically advanced scientific research results, and strive for international advanced level results, must be rated and accepted by higher authorities. Municipal laboratories are basically similar to provincial laboratories..*

Since it is an innovative country, technological innovation achievements should be at the international leading level in order to be competitive and creative.

The establishment of high-tech laboratories and national key laboratories should encourage the opening of new research fields. Innovative countries should establish state-level high-tech laboratories, open up high-tech research centers in new fields, and strive for strong government support and scientific development.

Therefore, in order to build an innovative country and build a scientific and technological innovation center, we must first vigorously build a laboratory to make talents useful and to make the product a place of scientific research and innovation; to make talents have a place to cultivate; to enable graduate students to cultivate experimental sites; to make the professors of colleges and universities have innovation, achievements, and masters. The construction of laboratories should be vigorously popularized, and scientific and technological innovations should be made to make the national central city a national science and technology innovation center.

Therefore, the construction of an innovative country, the construction of scientific and technological innovation center, must first vigorously build the laboratory, so that talent can make use of the product; scientific research and innovation of the land; so that people have to cultivate the land; so that graduate students have cultivated experimental areas; College professors have innovation, a result, a master of the land.

5. The objectives of the scientific and technological innovation:

1). *Production of the innovative results*

It should produce the achievement and produce the main innovation results or achievement with competition and creation;

And strive to generate the original innovation results, original results;

It should produce the product and the a new industry and product the new enterprise with the combination of production and learning and research

2). *Production of talent and production of a high-tech talent and production of the science and technology leading talent and production of a master of science*

Talents should be both ability and moral, medicine is benevolence, and ethics is the first

Talents should be truly talented, with results, achievements, innovation and superb skills or talent should be true to learn, should be fruitful, successful, innovative and superb technology

3). The importance of basic research, basic research leads to new knowledge, it provides scientific capital, it creates a reserve of knowledge, new products and new processes are not one that is fully mature, they are built on new principle and new ideas. These new principles and new concepts have been painstakingly developed in scientific research work.

Basic research leads to new knowledge, which provides the capital of science, which creates a reserve of knowledge. New products and new processes are not completely mature at the first emergence. And these new principles and new ideas are developed hard in the scientific research work.

The development of science is based on the innovation of basic theory. This is a big scientific achievement. Discovering new theories, new laws, new doctrines, and new laws is a big innovation.

Scientific advancement relies on the emergence of new scientific knowledge that can only be obtained through basic research.

Basic research in medical science is very important for achieving progress in combating cancer. *Without a breakthrough in basic research, clinical efficacy is difficult to improve* or the fundamental research in medical science is very important to progress in the fight against cancer. If there is no breakthrough in basic research, the clinical efficacy is difficult to improve.

The government should encourage the opening of new research areas and conquer the cancer and develop new products and new industries and the new knowledge to achieve these tasks comes from basic scientific research.

I deeply understand the importance of basic research:

In 1985, I conducted a petition with more than 3,000 patients who underwent radical surgery for various cancers. It was found that most patients relapsed and metastasized 2 to 3 years after surgery, and some even metastasized several months after surgery. This made me realize that although the operation is successful, the long-term efficacy is not satisfactory. Postoperative recurrence and metastasis are the key factors affecting the long-term efficacy of the operation. Therefore, basic research must be carried out, so we established the Institute of Experimental Surgery and spent 24 years conducting basic research and clinical validation of a series of experimental studies from the following three aspects:

1 to explore the pathogenesis, invasion and recurrence, metastasis mechanism of cancer, and to find experimental research to regulate the effective measures of recurrence and metastasis;

2 to find new anti-cancer, anti-metastatic, anti-recurrence new drugs from natural medicine;

3 clinical validation work.

We conducted a basic experimental study of cancer onset, invasion, recurrence, and metastasis mechanisms in the laboratory for 4 years. After 3 years of experimental research from natural drugs, it was found a batch of XZ-C$_{1-10}$ immunomodulatory anticancer Chinese medicine, and then the clinical validation of more than 12,000 patients with advanced or postoperative metastatic cancer in 16 years; the application of XZ-c immunomodulation of anticancer traditional Chinese medicine has achieved good results. It can improve the quality of life of patients, improve their symptoms and significantly prolong their survival.

After the basic research of the above experimental research, from experiment to clinical, and from clinical to experimental the summary of experimental research and clinical verification data has risen to the theoretical sublimation and propose new discoveries.

New understanding and new theoretical insights:

(1) One of the causes and pathogenesis of cancer is thymus atrophy, impaired thymus function, and low immune function;

(2) Proposed the theoretical basis and experimental basis of XZ-immunomodulation therapy;

(3) To propose cancer treatment, update ideas, change concepts, and establish a comprehensive treatment concept;

(4) Initiative for the mode of multidisciplinary treatment of cancer treatment

The whole course of treatment is based on radical surgery, supplemented by biological immunity, traditional Chinese medicine, XZ-C immunoregulation, and differentiation induction. Short-course treatment is mainly based on radiotherapy and chemotherapy, and cannot be long-range or over-extended;

(5) Evaluation and questioning of systemic intravenous chemotherapy for solid cancer;

(6) Initiatives for reform, the physical cancer should be reformed as target organ intravascular chemotherapy;

(7) Proposed new concepts, new models, and new methods for cancer treatment;

(8) Three monographs have been published in 10 years:

1). "New understanding and new model of cancer treatment" published by Hubei Science and Technology in 2001;

2). "New concept and new method of cancer metastasis treatment" was published by the People's Military Medical Press in 2006. In April 2007, it was awarded the "Three Hundred" original publishing project certificate by the General Administration of the People's Republic of China;

3). "New Concepts and New Methods for Cancer Treatment" published in October 2011 by the People's Military Medical Press. Later, Dr. Bin Wu, an American medical scientist, translated it into English. The English version was published in USA on March 26, 2013, and is distributed internationally.

In summary, experimental research and basic research are very important. Without experimental research and breakthroughs in basic research, clinical efficacy is difficult to improve, and it is difficult to propose new understandings, new concepts, and new theoretical insights. The laboratory is the key, I have a good laboratory, I am the director of the Institute of Experimental Surgery, and also the director of clinical surgery so that the experimental research and basic research and clinical validation are easy to take care of.

6. *The scientific and technological innovation and the timely transformation of development results is the key. The achievements of scientific and technological innovation should be transformed, developed and applied in a timely manner to benefit the people.*

One of the purposes of technological innovation is to produce innovative results. With results, inspection and acceptance should be identified. It conducts results identification through the results appraisal meeting or the results council and through the results level rating acceptance. The original innovation results should be verified.

The project does not equal the results - some universities currently promote, promote, and recruit graduate students, all attach importance to the project. This is okay, but this understanding is not enough because the project does not equal the outcome. With the project, it is not necessarily the result. Only when the project has achieved results, it just represents the academic level and scientific research achievements.

At present, some research institutes of colleges and universities only attach importance to scientific research projects and funds, and do not attach importance to the acceptance of scientific research results. A large number of projects have not yet achieved scientific research results, and they have ended up. The state puts a large amount of research funds into colleges and universities every year. The scientific research department must cherish it very much. It is necessary to obtain corresponding results. It should be strictly implemented, and the results will be submitted, the identification and acceptance of scientific research results will be carried out, and the particles will be returned to the warehouse. To achieve the acceptance of scientific research results and the rating of results, the research office is full of vitality, innovation every year, and fruitful results.

Research Office should pay attention to the acceptance of scientific research, particle sweeping warehouse.

How to evaluate research results?

There should be a certificate or certificate of government research results.

There should be a scientific research achievement certificate or a scientific and technological research result report.

There should be academic research results or research papers of the above projects in academic conferences at home and abroad and academic influence at home and abroad.

Or research papers are published in magazines, or the research monographs are published.

Scientific research results should be timely transformation and development.

What if I have scientific research results?

It must be transformed and developed into practicality to benefit people and society, and should not be "high-pitch or high-court". It should not be locked in "deep squat" and should be transformed and developed in time.

After appraised or reviewed the acquired scientific research results, It's not a good idea to put it on the "high-shelf "or locked in "deep squat", it should go down the high court, go out of the squat, carry out transformation, development, application and produce social and economic benefits and serve the society.

How to transform scientific and technological achievements? This has been a big problem for many years. It is an unsolved big problem in the country. But this is a problem that must be studied and discussed.

A scientific and technological innovation is a great waste if it is not transformed, developed and applied in time to benefit the people.

When an innovative country is built and a scientific and technological innovation center is formed, it will inevitably result in scientific and technological achievements. It will be springing up and flourishing, and will be full of scientific research results and a bumper harvest every year.

What should I do after the harvest of these scientific and technological achievements? Is it stacked in the storage room? Is it the "high cabinet"? Is it locked in "squat"? How to do?

It should be transformed and developed and applied in time to benefit the society and to benefit the people and it develops science and the social progresses and people are happy.

Innovative countries have prospered technological innovation and scientific research achievement is huge.

How to convert? and how to develop? and how to apply? it becomes the key.

For the transformation of results, development is the key. This issue must be put on the agenda in time to establish a transformation mechanism for results and to establish a results transformation agency and to make the results work and to generate social and economic benefits.

At present, many professors in colleges and universities in China have scientific research results or quasi-results. I have a series of results in hand. There are no intermediaries, no brokers, no ones to match the bridge, I don't know how to attract investment. There are no mechanisms and institutions for the transformation and development of scientific research results. I don't know what level of government to ask for guidance and support. Scientists and researchers have achieved results in hand and there is no method to be used and no one cares, and it is put in the "high cabinet"; entrepreneurs want results, can't find them, can't get them. This is currently a pair of the prominent social contradiction.

How to do? I want to make a suggestion:

Government-led, Match line or connect line and set up the bridge or Bypass,

Government-led, attract the business to invest the capital;

There are job fairs in the talent market or talent market recruitment. Scientific research results should also have results presentations and the achievement results fair and the presentation of results and inviting investment.

Through government-led, it is to establish a committee for the transformation and development of scientific research achievements. Under the leading position it sets up the achievement or results transformation Work Center and Conversion Office and it establishes a conversion work mechanism and a conversion work organization. The Chamber of Commerce is selling products and the achievement or results meeting are the result promotion and intermediary.

In short:

How to build an innovative country and national Science and Technology Innovation Center?

I think talents and laboratories are the key. With innovation results, the transformation of results is the key.

Talent ----a laboratory----a scientific and technological innovation results -----the transformation and development of the results

1. Talents must be true and practical or the talent personnel must be genuine talent, practical, and must be both ability and moral

How to evaluate and confirm that there is real talent?

It must have gained scientific research results or have academic achievements. I am an old doctor and senior professor who has been a doctor for 55 years so that I am thinking about medical ethics which should be: the medicine is benevolence, the ethics first or the moral is for the first or the virtue is the first.

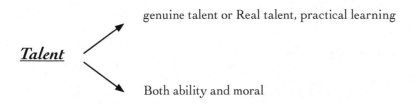

Talent
genuine talent or Real talent, practical learning
Both ability and moral

Leading talents in scientific research must preside over national-level research projects and obtain scientific research results at the international advanced level or domestic leading level, and more mature research experience.

2. *The laboratory is an incubator for technological innovation. The laboratory is an incubator for the training of scientific research personnel*.

Without a laboratory, it is impossible to produce scientific and technological fruits. Without a laboratory, it is difficult to produce scientific and technological talents. Without high-quality laboratory equipment, modern high-tech innovations cannot be produced. Masters Yang Zhenning and Ding Yuzhong are awarded the Nobel Prize in Physics through well-equipped laboratories.

3. *With the achievements of scientific and technological innovation, timely transformation and development and application are the key.*

Innovative countries have built science and technology innovation centers, and the results of independent innovation or original innovation are numerous. *How to transform, develop and apply in time to benefit the people? How to combine the science, industry, trade and production, learning, research, matching line and building the bridges to further develop prosperity and innovation?*

It must be put on the agenda, establish a transformation mechanism for results, and establish a transformation mechanism for results.

Therefore it is recommended that:

The government is leading, setting up provincial and municipal scientific research achievements transformation and development work committees, setting up a results transformation work center and research work transformation work office, and establishing a transformation mechanism and transformation institution.

We should vigorously build science and technology laboratories. The gap between our universities and European and American universities is mainly because of their high-tech laboratories. There are fewer high-tech universities in China.

I think: How to build an innovative country?

Talents and laboratories are the key.

The purpose of scientific and technological innovation is *to produce innovative results*.

Innovative countries should make major breakthroughs in scientific research in key areas, and innovation achievements in several fields enters the forefront of the world.

How to solve the problem of combining science and technology with economics, the transformation of scientific research achievements?

The exploration and development are the key. This issue must be put on the agenda in a timely manner. It must be led by the government, establish a transformation mechanism for results, establish a transformation system or institution for results. Through the Office of Achievement Transformation, combine scientists with entrepreneurs to carry out results transformation and development and make scientific research results play a role and produce or generate economic and social benefits.

I will now list talents → labs → results → transformation and conversion and development. The list of the benign relationships is shown below:

The Figureof The Relationship of Talent → Labs → Results of the Relationship

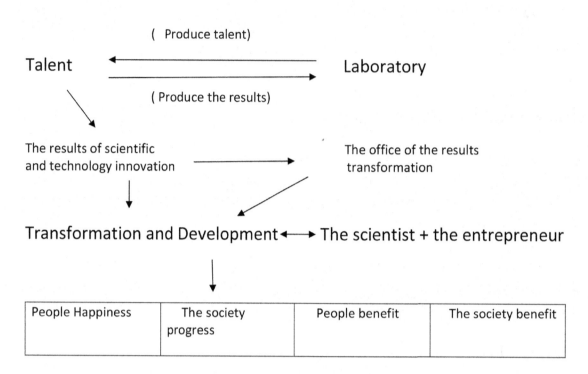

People Happiness	The society progress	People benefit	The society benefit

八

The Strategic thinking and advice on conquering cancer

The Strategic Ideas and Suggestions on Conquering Cancer

At present cancer has become a major disease that seriously threatens human health, and its incidence is increasing at an annual rate of 3-5%. The number of morbidity and deaths increased by 24.7% and 19.2% respectively compared with 10 years ago. The traditional three major treatments, nearly a hundred years, the cancer patient mortality rate is still the first, what should I do? How is the research road to go? It should be analyzed and reflected and studied.

Where is the direction of the road to victory over cancer?

- Professor Xu Ze (XU ZE) believes that the road is in scientific research, and the road is in the scientific research on the prevention and treatment of cancer; the road is exploring the experimental basis of the etiology, pathogenesis and pathophysiology of cancer; the road is studying the whole process of cancer occurrence and development; the road is to reform and develop the traditional therapy; the road is in multidisciplinary research; the road is studying the prevention and treatment of cancer metastasis and recurrence; the road is in the study of "three early".

Through the scientific research on the prevention and treatment of cancer through the road, human beings will surely overcome cancer, and will eventually conquer cancer.

How to conquer cancer I see one:

1. *The road to scientific research is the experimental basic research to explore the cause of cancer, pathogenesis, pathophysiology*

1). I believe that the development of cancer science research is the urgent need of the current status of tumor disciplines, we must recognize what the problems of the status of cancer disciplines are, how to do?

Although cancer treatment has been going on for more than a century, it has now entered the second decade of the 21st century. However, "oncology" is still a backward discipline in various medical sciences. Why? It is because the etiology, pathogenesis, pathophysiology of "oncology" are not well understood. The oncology discipline is still a scientific virgin for scientific research, and it needs a lot of basic scientific research and clinical basic research. Although the traditional three major treatments (surgery, radiotherapy, chemotherapy) have been applied for nearly a hundred years, thousands of cancer patients have undergone radiotherapy and chemotherapy. But what is the result, the cancer mortality rate so far is still the first cause of death for urban and rural residents in China. How should the road go? It should be deeply introspected, in-depth analysis, and in-depth study.

Why is this so? The main reasons are:

(1) the etiology of cancer is not clear, the pathogenesis is unclear, pathophysiology is not clear, there are a lot of basic theoretical problems which are not clear.

(2) the biological characteristics and biological behavior of cancer cells still lack sufficient understanding.

(3) the molecular mechanism of cancer cell metastasis still lacks sufficient understanding.

(4) the occurrence and development and cloning and proliferation, invasion, metastasis, planting, complex biological behavior of cancer are still lack of understanding which all are subject to conditional units for research.

The current cancer treatment program is still quite blind. Diagnosis means are behind and once the cancer is found, the cancer is already in the middle and late stage and the treatment effect is poor. Because the cause and the pathogenesis and the pathophysiology are still lack of adequate understanding and did not carry out the full experimental study of basic research, the current understanding of the tumor discipline seems still not clear enough fuzzy state or hazy state and the knowledge of the tumor is still in a very backward state.

Many large-scale tumor hospital or university affiliated hospital have not established cancer laboratory, cannot carry out the basic research of cancer, nor the establishment of cancer animal laboratory, can not be carried out animal model test. Anti-cancer metastasis and recurrence must be carried out in the basic model of cancer animal model and it should be used in nude mice to establish a variety of cancer animal models to study the transfer of cancer cells and the mechanism. (My experimental surgery laboratory with the removal of mouse thymus to produce bearing-cancer animal model 60 times, 7 years, with pure mice Kunming mice to replace the establishment of animal model of about 10,000 animals)

Why is it paid attention to the basic research laboratory? It is because if there is no basic research breakthrough, the clinical efficacy is difficult to improve.

2). The experimental surgery is a key to open the medical restricted area.

Experimental surgery is extremely important in the development of medical science. It is a key to open the medical exclusion zone. The pathogenesis and prevention methods of many diseases have been studied in countless animal experiments, and the stability results have been applied to the clinic to promote the development of the medical cause and to improve medical quality and develop new prevention methods

Our laboratory of experimental surgery was established in May 1980. Under the auspices of Professor Xu Ze, the experimental study and pathological study of cirrhotic refractory ascites were performed.

Experimental study on the pathology, pathophysiology and pathogenesis of schistosomiasis japonicum was investigated by experimental surgical methods; Experimental study on the pathogenesis of schistosomiasis cirrhosis with portal hypertension was studied. National and provincial scientific research projects, such as the experimental study of hepatocytes transplanted into the spleen to form the second liver to treat liver failure, have a certain foundation for experimental research.

In early 1987, this laboratory began to turn to the experimental tumor research. Researchers have carried out the transplantation of cancer cells, built experimental tumor animal models, explored the pathogenesis and pathophysiology of tumor, and investigated the law and mechanism of cancer cell metastases in cancer-bearing animal models and changes of the host's immune function. And then researchers have discussed Chinese herbal medicines with good anti-cancer effects, made a strict and scientific screening study of Chinese herbal medicines with anti-cancer and cancer inhibited effect in vivo of cancer-bearing animal models. In order to develop the career of cancer prevention and treatment, researchers commit themselves to the experimental researches of exploring the cause, pathogenesis and pathophysiology of cancer and further extracting Chinese herbal medicines with the effect of cancer prevention and cure.

With the practical requirement in our college's medical science situation, Institute of Experimental Surgery of Hubei College of Traditional Chinese Medicine was set up in March 1991 on the basis of experimental surgical laboratory. Professor Xu Ze serves as director of the institute and Academician Qiu Fazu is invited as the mentor. *Their research target and task are: Institute of Experimental Surgery is mainly to tackle key problems of cancer. The emphasis is to adopt the method of experimental surgery to carry out fundamental researches of experimental tumors and control researches of clinical patients*. This research laboratory of experimental tumor adopts biological engineering technology and genetic engineering technology of cancer cells, exploits the fundamental research and clinical practice of tumor biological therapy and immunization therapy, develops and promotes the career of cancer prevention and treatment.

3). In our laboratory it has been found the following understandings from the experimental tumor research.

(1) Our laboratory can make a tumor-bearing animal model by removing the thymus (Thymus, TH) from mice. Injection of immunosuppressive agents can also contribute to the establishment of cancer-bearing animal models. The conclusions of the study prove that the occurrence and development of cancer have a significant relationship with the thymus and its function of the host immune organs. Or the research results indicate that there is an obvious link between the generation and growth of cancer and the host's immune organ- thymus and its function.

(2) When we explore the effect of tumor on the immune organs of the body, it was found that as the cancer progressed, the thymus showed progressive atrophy (600 tumor-bearing animal model mice), and the host thymus showed acute progressive atrophy after inoculation of cancer cells. That is to say, the host's thymus presents acute progressive atrophy after inoculation of cancer cells.

(3) It was also found through experiments that some of the experimental mice were not successfully vaccinated, or the tumors grew very small, and the thymus

did not shrink significantly. In order to understand the relationship between tumor and thymus atrophy, we removed a group of experimental mice when the transplanted solid tumor grew to the size of the thumb. After 1 month, the thymus was found to have no progressive atrophy. Therefore, we speculate that a solid tumor may produce a factor that is not known to inhibit the thymus, which needs further study.

(4) The above experimental results prove that:

Progression of the tumor can cause progressive atrophy of the thymus. So, can we use some methods to prevent the host thymus from shrinking? Therefore, we further designed and wanted to find ways or drugs to prevent thymocyte atrophy in tumor-bearing mice through animal experiments. Therefore, we used this immune organ cell transplantation to restore the experimental function of the immune organ. We are investigating the atrophy of the thymus gland in the immune system to stop the progression of the tumor, and to find ways to restore the function of the thymus and reconstitute the immune system. The mice were transplanted with fetal liver cells, fetal spleen cells and fetal thymus cells, and the immune function of the recipients was reconstructed. The results show: The S, T, and L groups were transplanted together (200 experimental mice), and the tumor regression rate was 40%. The complete regression rate of long-term tumors was 46.67%. Long-term survival of patients have the complete tumor regression

4). *From the experimental research results, it was proposed one of the causes and pathogenesis of cancer may be thymus atrophy and immune dysfunction*.

Our laboratory has conducted a series of animal experiments on the etiology, pathogenesis and pathophysiology of cancer. Analyze and think from the results of experimental research, so that we can obtain new discoveries, new ideas, and new inspirations: One of the causes of cancer may be thymus atrophy, impaired thymus function, and low immune function. Therefore, Professor Xu Ze (XU ZE) first proposed the cause and mechanism of cancer in the world. It may be atrophy of the thymus, impaired central immune function, low immune function, decreased immune surveillance and immune escape. But what is the cause of the host's thymus atrophy? The author repeatedly thinks about speculation: It is possible that a solid tumor will produce a factor to inhibit the Thymus, which needs further study. We can call it "the cancer suppressor factor for Thymus". Or A series of animal experimental studies have been done for exploring the cause, pathogenesis and pathophysiology of cancer.

The analysis and think of experimental results produce new discovery, new thinking and new revelation. That is, one of cancer causes may be the atrophy of thymus, the damage of thymus function and the hypo-function of immune organs. Therefore, Professor Xu Ze first proposes the idea in the world that one of cancer causes and pathogeneses may be the atrophy of thymus, the function damage of central immune organs, the hypo-function of immune organs, the reduction of immune surveillance function and immunologic escape. But what leads to the host's thymus atrophy? The writer ruminates over this question and speculates that the solid tumor might produce a kind of factor that can suppress thymus; nevertheless, the speculation needs further experimental researches. This kind of factor is temporarily <u>called "thymus suppressor cancer-factor"</u>.

5). Subsequently, the writer raises XZ-C immunologic regulation and control therapy------ the theoretical and experimental basis of "thymus protection for enhancing immunity; pulp protection for hemogenesis" in XZ-C immunologic regulation and control therapy. Or Later, it proposed XZ-C immunomodulation therapy - the theoretical basis and experimental basis for protection of Thymus and Increase of immune function and protection of hemogenesis in XZ-C immunologic mediation and control therapy.

Based on the inspiration from the above experimental results about the cause and pathogenesis of cancer, the new theory and new method of XZ-C immunologic mediation and control targeted therapy that first proposed by Professor Xu Ze have their theoretical and experimental basis. Our presented therapeutic principle and theory of "thymus protection for enhancing immunity; pulp protection for hemogenesis" are reasonable and scientific. Through sixteen years' clinical observation of over 12,000 patients with intermediate- or advanced-stage cancer in Twilight Specialist Out-patient Department, it can clearly show that this therapeutic principle with more than 30 years' clinical application is correct and reasonable. The therapeutic effectiveness is satisfactory and trusted by patients.

As an old saying goes, "Once the headrope of fishing net is pulled up, all its meshes open." As long as the thymus atrophy might be one of cancer causes and pathogeneses, then theoretical basis of therapy must emerge at its proper moment.

6). Review the history of cancer etiology in the past 100 years

*In the history of medicine, more than 2500 years ago, the scholar of ancient Greek-**Hippocrates** used a word "**Cancer**" to describe tumor. From then on people started the study and* *understanding of malignant tumor. Or In the history of medical development, as early as more than 2,500 years ago, the ancient Greek scholar Hippocrates used the term "Cancer" to describe the tumor, and people began to study and understand the malignant tumor disease.*

*Until 1775, British doctor found that boys **who sweep air flue for a long time are easy to suffer from carcinoma of scrotum.** Then this doctor proposed the theory that the production of tumor is **closely related to environmental factor. Until** 1775, British doctors discovered that boys who had long cleaned the flue were susceptible to scrotal cancer, and proposed a theory that tumors are closely related to environmental factors.*

*In the late 19ᵗʰ, German doctor discovered that workers who touch dye have an impressively high proportion of **suffering from bladder carcinoma.** Afterwards some chemical substances successfully induce tumor in animals; tobacco components exert an influence on **lung cancer; Aspergillus flavus has a definite relation with liver cancer. All these have provided direct evidences for the theory of cancer caused by chemical substances.** Or, in the late 19ᵗʰ century, German doctors found that workers exposed to dyes had an abnormally high **rate of bladder cancer.** Later, some chemicals induced tumor success in animals. The effects of tobacco ingredients have **effects on lung cancer.** The relationship between Aspergillus flavus and **liver cancer** provides a direct basis for the theory of chemical substances to cancer.*

In 1908, Danish pathologists Ellerman and Bang discovered that chicken leukemia can be transmitted to healthy chickens through cell-free Shanghai liquid. Two years later, American pathologist Rous proved that a sarcoma of chicken is caused **by a virus and establishes the theory of viral carcinogenesis.** Or in 1908, Danish pathologist Ellerman and Bang found that chicken's leukemia can pass to healthy chickens through the filtered solution without cells. Two years later, American pathologist Rous proved that a kind of sarcoma in chicken is caused by virus, **which establishes the theory of oncogenic virus.**

The relation between human tumor and virus was established after EB virus was found in Burkitt lymphoma in 1964. The following researches show that EB virus and nasopharyngeal carcinoma, hepatitis b virus and primary carcinoma of liver, human papilloma virus and cervical carcinoma have an intimate relation. Those all lay a solid foundation for the theory of oncogenic virus. Or **The relationship between human tumors and viruses was established in 1964 after the discovery of EB virus in Burkitt's lymphoma.** Since then, studies have shown that EB virus has **a close relationship with nasopharyngeal carcinoma, hepatitis B virus and primary liver cancer, human papilloma virus and cervical cancer, which have laid a solid foundation for viral carcinogenesis.**

__People's awareness of the cause of cancer continues to expand__. When it is found that the sea cancer of the seamen who are often exposed to the sun is very high, *__the physical factors are considered to cause cancer__*. It was not until people induced tumors in rats *__after high-dose X-ray irradiation__* that people began to confirm the *__theory of physical carcinogenesis__*. In the 1940s, after the atomic bombing of Hiroshima and Nagasaki in Japan, the incidence of various *__tumors and leukemias among__* survivors was significantly increased. In the course of clinical cancer treatment, iatrogenic leukemia occurs after the primary lesion is controlled, and these facts provide evidence for the physical carcinogenesis theory. Or, People's knowledge of tumor causes continues to expand. Finding that sailors who often expose to the sun have a high risk of contracting skin carcinoma, people start to consider physical factors which may cause cancer. Until discovering that rate tumor can be induced after a large dosage of X-irradiation, people begin to confirm the theory of cancer caused by physical factors. In 1940s, after the explosion of atomic bombs in Japanese cities of Hiroshima and Nagasaki, various tumors and leukemias in survivors occur in high incidence. In the process of clinical cancer therapy, iatrogenic leukemia appears after the primary lesion is controlled. The two facts provide evidences for the theory of cancer caused by physical factors.

__Although people have a preliminary understanding of the etiology of tumors, the pathogenesis and pathophysiology of malignant tumors are still not clear, and there is no effective prevention and treatment. Therefore, it is urgent to conduct extensive, in-depth and subtle research on the pathogenesis, pathophysiology and control measures of tumors__. Or. although having had a preliminary knowledge of the tumor etiology, people still feel indefinite about the pathogenesis and pathophysiology of malignant tumor, and also lack effective preventive and therapeutic measures. Therefore, it is urgently necessary to have an extensive, in-depth and detailed study of tumor's pathogenesis and pathophysiology as well as prophylactic-therapeutic measures.

The above review of the history of cancer in the past 100 years, the cause of cancer, pathogens, pathogenesis, pathophysiology research is still very few, so far cancer is not a disease is still unclear.Because according to the definition of a disease, there must be pathogens, etiology, pathogenesis, pathophysiology, and pathology. However, in the past 100 years, people have been striving for clinical research and clinical basic research in surgery, radiotherapy, chemotherapy, and laboratory research and clinical research on the mutation, cloning, proliferation, invasion, metastasis, and breeding of cancer cells. Basic research, such as invasion, metastasis, cancer thrombus, immunity, endocrine, virus, etc., is rarely done. Exploring the etiology, pathogenesis, pathophysiology, metastasis, and recurrence of cancer must be carried out in the basic research of cancer-bearing animal models. Rats have established various animal models of cancer to study the laws and mechanisms of cancer cell invasion and metastasis. Or, reviewing the above research history of cancer over the past one hundred years, we can find that researches about cancer's cause, pathogeny, pathogenesis and pathophysiology are still quite rare. Until now whether or not cancer is a kind of disease can hardly be explained. That's because according to the definition, a disease must have the pathogeny, cause, pathogenesis, pathophysiology and pathology. But for one hundred years, people have always applied themselves to clinical and clinical fundamental researches of surgical operation, radiotherapy and chemotherapy. But in aspects of regular laboratory fundamental and clinical fundamental researches of cancer cell mutation, clone, proliferation, invasion, metastasis and implantation, people have done a little, such as invasion, metastasis, cancer embolus, immunization, endocrine and virus, etc. **Exploring cancer's cause, pathogenesis, pathophysiology, metastasis and relapse must depend on the fundamental research of cancer-bearing animal models. All sorts of cancer animal models should be built with nude mice, in order to study the law and mechanism of cancer cells' invasions and metastases.**

How to overcome the cancer I see two:

2. The road of scientific research is to study the occurrence and the development of the whole process of prevention and treatment of cancer

1) Xu Ze (XU ZE) on the idea, strategy, planning diagram of conquering cancer

How to fight cancer

↓

Where is the road?

↓

Our ideas, strategies, experience should be divided into three parts

↓

Before the formation of cancer---- for the prevention part -------anti-mutation

↓

There may be malignant tendencies of precancerous lesions------ for the intervention part

↓

Has been the treatment of primary cancer and the treatment of anti-metastatic part

2) The way-out of cancer treatment is in the "three early", the way out of anti-cancer is to prevent

If we can treat well in precancerous or early stage cancer, the number of patients who progress to invasion and metastasis will decrease, which will reduce the incidence of cancer. Therefore, we believe that the current local cancer hospitals are mainly for the treatment of patients with advanced disease, even if the treatment results are good, they can only reduce the mortality rate. While neglecting the stage of susceptibility, precancerous lesions, early patients, it is impossible to reduce the incidence of cancer. Therefore, we believe that we must pay attention to the whole process of cancer occurrence and development. After all this is the real global change of strategic importance.

We have been doing tumor surgery for many years. The more patients are treated, the higher the incidence of cancer is. This makes me realize that cancer should not only pay attention to treatment, but also pay attention to prevention, so as to stop at the source. Cancer treatment is in the "three early" (early detection, early diagnosis, early treatment). The way to fight cancer is prevention.

If patients have been treated well in the stage of precancerous lesion or early stage, then the number of patients in middle or advanced stage of invasion and metastasis will fall off. Thus, the cancer incidence rate will also decline. Therefore, we hold that the present tumor hospitals in various places mainly focus on the cancer treatment in middle or advanced stage. Even though the therapeutic result is effective, it can only bring the reduction of cancer mortality rate. But if ignoring the stage of susceptibility, precancerous lesion or early stage, it will be impossible to reduce the cancer incidence rate. Therefore, we must put much emphasis on the whole process of cancer production and growth.

As stated above, the strategic center of gravity of tumor treatment and prevention moves forward. ***There are two aspects in its meaning.***

One is to prevent cancer by changing life style and improving environmental pollution;

The other is to cure precancerous lesion for inhibiting cancer's development to the invasion stage, middle stage or advanced stage.

In 1990, our institute's specialist out-patient department of tumor surgery once opened the outpatient service of "three kinds of earliness" to carry out various endoscopies and biopsies, through which have found many atypical hyperplasia of stomach, intestinal metaplasia, atrophic gastritis and hyperplasia of mammary glands, etc. These "precancerous lesions" are difficult to treat. Then how to handle these precancerous lesions or precancerous conditions so as to prevent their cancerations urgently needs clinical researches to look for better treatment methods.

3) It should pay attention to the diagnosis and technology research of the basis and clinics of precancerous lesions.

The key to cancer treatment is in the "three early", and how to deal with precancerous lesions is a critical stage of cancer prevention and treatment.

The present cancer diagnosis mainly depends on image examinations of type-B ultrasonic, CT and MRI. But as soon as the cancer comes to light, it has reached the middle or advanced stage. Many patients have lost the chance of radical excision. Although the complex treatment has been done, the therapeutic effects are still poor. If the cancer is in the early stage or belongs to the carcinoma in situ, then the curative effect of operation will be better and the cancer can be cured. Therefore, the cancer treatment should strive for "three kinds of earliness", which refers to early detection, early diagnosis and early treatment.

Because cancer's pathogenic factors are not very clear, the primary prevention is still quite difficult.

Studies in recent years indicate that malignant tumor rarely has a direct carcinomatous change in normal tissues. Before the occurrence of tumor in clinical diagnosis, cancer often goes through quite a long evolution stage, which is the stage of precancerous lesion. Early identification and control of these precancerous lesions will bring positive significances for the secondary prevention of cancer.

What is precancerous lesion?

The precancerous lesion is a histopathology concept, which refers to a kind of tissues with the dysplasia of cells or a type of cell dysplasia that is a precancerous lesion. Precancerous lesion has the potential to become cancerous. If there is no cure in a long period, precancerous lesion will evolve into cancer or it may turn into cancer. In other words, precancerous lesion just has the possibility of changing into cancer. That is to say, precancerous lesions only have the possibility of turning into cancer. But not all the precancerous lesions will eventually become cancer. Through proper treatments, precancerous lesions may return to their normal states or have a spontaneous regression. If properly treated, it may return to normal or naturally resolve.

Canceration is a developing process with several stages. There is a stage of precancerous lesion between normal cells and cancer. It is a slow process from precancerous lesion evolving into cancer, which needs many years or even more than ten years. It is closely related to The length of canceration course and the strength of carcinogenic factors and individual susceptibility and immunologic function. Therefore, the study of precancerous lesion is of great importance to cancer's prevention and control.

How to overcome the cancer I see the three:

3. The road to scientific research lies in the development of multidisciplinary research and the special in-depth basic and clinical research

1). Oncology research is the most complex and difficult subject in medical research. It involves multidisciplinary knowledge and theory, including pathology, cytology, immunology, virology, molecular biology, medical genetics, immunopharmacology, molecular oncology. Studying the pathogenesis of tumors at the molecular level and understanding the cause of the disease thereby provide intervention and treatment for effective prevention and treatment of tumors.

The present surgical operation is still the most important, frequently used, definite and effective therapeutic methods to treat malignant tumor. But relapse or metastasis often appears in the short or long term after surgical operation. Follow-up results of more than 3,000 patients who have accepted cancer surgeries of chest and abdomen discover that postoperative relapse and metastasis are key factors for long-term therapeutic effectiveness of surgical operation. Therefore, an issue is raised that the method and measure of preventing and treating postoperative relapse and metastasis are important for improving long-term therapeutic effectiveness. There is a must to carry out fundamental and clinical interdisciplinary study on resisting relapse and metastasis.

Since 1970s, in view of extremely high recurrence and metastatic rate after cancer operation, in order to prevent postoperative recurrence and metastasis, patients accept a series of adjuvant chemotherapies. Some patients have even started to accept preoperative chemotherapies, but the results are not fully up to expectations. Postoperative relapse and metastasis still come out in a short time. How to prevent recurrence and resist metastasis to get a good long-term effect is the matter that really deserves clinicians' serious and objective analysis, reflection, consider and study.

Now in the early 21st century, cancer recurrence and metastasis have become the "bottleneck" in cancer treatment. The main problem of cancer treatment still focuses on how to fight against metastasis. If not solving the metastasis after radical operation of cancer, cancer treatment cannot have a further improvement. We hold that tackling key cancer problem mainly depends on the resistance to metastasis. The key problem of cancer treatment is to tackle metastasis and recurrence.

2). *Organize multi-disciplinary joint researches with large-scale cooperation among hospitals.*

Therefore, it is necessary to carry out basic and clinical research on anti-cancer metastasis and recurrence, and carry out joint research on multidisciplinary and multi-hospital cooperation. Organize scientific research collaborations in provinces, municipal colleges and universities, hospitals, hospitals, specialist hospitals, professors, experts, scholars, doctors, masters, hospitals, doctors, and anti-cancer people. Take the road of large-scale cooperation and joint research, promote scientific research cooperation, attach importance to the organization of scientific research and technical strength, and enrich the anti-cancer scientific and technological forces of anti-cancer, anti-metastasis and recurrence. Or It is a must to carry out fundamental and clinical studies on resisting relapse and metastasis as well as multi-disciplinary joint researches with large-scale cooperation among hospitals. Organize professors, experts, scholars, doctors, master, and physicians in universities and colleges as well as their affiliated hospitals, independent hospitals and special hospitals on the level of Hubei province or Wuhan city and anti-cancer persons with lofty ideals to carry out research cooperation and walk the way of joint researches with large-scale cooperation. Advocate large-scale research cooperation, pay attention to organize scientific and technical force of each side and raise anti-cancer force on resisting cancer, metastasis and relapse.

Anti-cancer research needs to involve multiple disciplines, not only clinical medicine, but also many marginal disciplines, interdisciplinary and basic disciplines. Cancer metastasis and recurrence studies include internal medicine, surgery, radiation, endocrine, drugs, immunity, molecular biology, viruses, biological information, genetic engineering, life sciences, molecular chemistry, mold chemistry, environmental protection, traditional Chinese medicine, and laboratory. Our city has the talents of the above disciplines and has a certain foundation. We can organize all kinds of scientific and technological strengths, work together, and take the road of scientific research and cooperation to jointly improve the level of anti-cancer metastasis and recurrence, and benefit the millions of cancer patients.

In order to overcome cancer and do anti-cancer research, basic and clinical research on the recurrence of cancer metastasis must be carried out and it is to conduct multi-disciplinary and multi-hospital cooperation and joint research.

It is necessary to establish the Wuhan Anticancer Research Association..

With the energetic support of academician Qiu Fazu, through the declaration and preparation of Xu Ze, Li Huiqiao and other professors, upon the local tax authorities' approval, they finally set up Wuhan anti-cancer institute on June 21, 2009. Then they establish a special committee for treating cancer metastasis and relapse, also organize academic and research team of tackling cancer metastasis to carry out academic research, academic discuss and academic propaganda, and open academic workshop or seminar. Thu they have trained many batches of senior talented young and middle-aged people on the study and treatment of resisting cancer metastasis for our province and city.

__The goal in anti-cancer study relies on "research". Under the guidance of scientific outlook on development, take the view angle of development and innovative spirit, focus__ *on the front sight and look into the future to develop medical science, research into the cancer prevention and control, the generation and growth of cancer, the pathogenesis of cancer metastasis relapse as well as the prevention and treatment of cancer. The research line is to discover, raise, study, solve or explain the problem.*

3). **Assemble the following professional research groups which are closely related to cancer; deeply specialize in fundamental and clinical discipline researches**.

In view of oncology study ranging over multi-disciplinary knowledge and theories, the related personnel must assemble relevant professional research groups to further specialize in and reply on the known knowledge and medical science in this subject, study and explore the unknown knowledge and future medical science in this subject, borderline subjects and interdisciplinary subjects to help conquer cancer. The following professional research groups should be set up. In the future, new subjects, interdisciplinary subjects or new industries may come out.

(1). Immunity and cancer research group:

In the modern history of tumor treatment, surgical operation, chemotherapy and radiotherapy are basic treatment methods. They have made some progress, but the whole curative effects are still not fully up to expectations. Cancer still occupies the number one in human causes of death.

The modern immunological therapy of malignant tumor began in the early 1970s. Through decades of unremitting efforts, with the development of technology, different treatment methods and drugs, such *as interferon, interleukin and LAK cells* appear in succession and have also got certain curative effects. But the successful application of *anti-CD20 monoclonal antibody (rituximab)* in lymphoid tumor just truly realizes immunization therapy and also opens up a new tumor therapeutic area——immune targeted therapy.

The earlier chapters in this book have already made some introductions. After four-year experimental research history of exploring pathogenic factors, pathogenesis and pathophysiology with cancer-bearing animal models, *our laboratory have found that removal of mouse's thymus can make cancer-bearing animal model; injecting immunosuppressant can also contribute to the buildup of cancer-bearing animal model and with the gradual growth of cancer, thymus presents progressive atrophy. Therefore, Professor Xu Ze first proposes the idea in the world that one of cancer causes and pathogeneses may be the atrophy of thymus, the function damage of thymus and the reduction of immune function. He also raises theoretical basis and experimental evidence of new theory and method——XZ-C targeted therapy of immune regulation and control.*

The latest clinical research task of immunity and cancer research group should be:

① to assess the condition of immunologic function in cancer patients;

② to monitor the curative effect of immune regulation therapy in cancer patients;

③to quantitatively measure the condition of immunologic function in radiotherapy and chemotherapy patients.

(2). The virus and cancer research group

Some of the cancer is known to be closely related to the virus, the treatment should be considered the appropriate treatment measures.

The etiology of certain cancerous tumors

As early as 1908 and 1911, people have found in succession that *leukemia cells of chicken and filtering medium of chicken sarcoma* can *induce leukemia and sarcoma*. In 1951, *leukemia virus* is found in mice. In the recent ten years, due to the rapid development of virology, immunology and molecular biochemistry, the study of tumor virus has also made fast progress. Thus it is confirmed one after the other that many viruses can induce tumor and even some human viruses (such as *adenovirus and herpes simplex virus*) can also induce the tumor of mouse. *EB virus* can induce the monkey's malignant tumor. Until now, only one quarter of over six hundred animal viruses are discovered to have the characteristic of causing tumor. Of special interest is chicken's Marek disease. It is a lymphoid tumor caused by chicken's simplex virus, which can lead to the mass mortality of chickens. Now this disease can be prevented with vaccine to get significant effect. Inspired by the important progress in the research of animal tumor virus, the research about virus pathogenesis of human tumor is also continuously developing. At present, it is discovered that some human tumors, such as *Burkitt lymphoid tumor, nasopharyngeal cancer, leukaemia, sarcoma, breast cancer and cervical carcinoma, are relevant to virus.*

(3). Hormone and cancer research group

*For some cancers known to be related **to hormones**, the carcinogenic factors should be further studied, and the hormones should be emphasized in the treatment. **In the prevention of cancer, we should pay attention to hormones and further study the existing knowledge**. Or, it is necessary to have a further study on the carcinogenic factors of some known cancers related to hormone. **Cancer treatment should lay stress on Hormone; while cancer prevention should pay attention to the further study of hormone based on the current knowledge**.*

Hormonal imbalance and tumor generation or Hormone imbalance and tumorigenesis

*Hormones are important chemicals that regulate the development and function of the body by neurohumoral fluids. Various hormones maintain a dynamic equilibrium relationship according to the law of the unity of opposites. In the case of a disease or some cause of endocrine disorders, certain hormones continue to act on sensitive tissues due to hormone imbalance, and this abnormal chronic stimulation may lead to cell proliferation and canceration. **A carcinogenic hormone refers to a hormone that promotes the growth of tissue cells, such as ovarian estrogen, pituitary gonadotropin, thyroid stimulating hormone, and prolactin.** In the case of breast cancer, in the absence of pituitary and ovarian hormones that promote breast growth, the breast is undeveloped, underdeveloped breast tissue is less prone to tumors, **so hormones are a necessary factor in the development of breast cancer**.*

*Experimental studies have shown that hormonal imbalance can induce tumors of the thyroid gland, anterior pituitary, ovary, testis, adrenal cortex, and accessory organs such as the uterus, cervix, vagina, and breast. It takes a long time for hormones to induce tumors and often need to have a certain genetic background and environmental factors as the disease conditions. In addition, hormones can also synergize with other carcinogenic factors, causing cancerous cells, or as a condition for other factors. Certain hormones such as Prostatic hormone have the effect of promoting cell differentiation and strengthening the immune response, and whether it has an effect on the carcinogenesis of cells when it is insufficiently secreted remains to be studied. Or in the case of a disease or some cause of endocrine disorders, certain hormones continue to act on sensitive tissues due to hormone imbalance, and this abnormal chronic stimulation may lead to cell proliferation and canceration. A carcinogenic hormone refers to a hormone that promotes the growth of tissue cells, such as ovarian estrogen, pituitary gonadotropin, thyroid stimulating hormone, and prolactin. Take breast cancer as an example. **In the absence of pituitary and ovarian hormones that promote breast growth, the breast is not developed, and the underdeveloped breast tissue is less prone to tumors. Hormone is therefore a necessary factor in the development of breast cancer.***

Experimental studies have shown that hormone disorders can induce tumors in the thyroid gland, anterior pituitary, ovary, testis, adrenal cortex, and accessory organs such as the uterus, cervix, vagina, and breast. Hormone-induced tumors take longer, and often require a certain genetic background and environmental factors as a disease condition; in addition, hormones can also synergize with other carcinogenic factors, causing cancerous cells, or as a condition of other factors. **<u>Certain hormones, such as prostate hormone, have the effect of promoting cell differentiation and strengthening the immune response</u>**, *and whether it affects the carcinogenesis of cells when the secretion is insufficient, remains to be studied.*

Or Hormone is an important chemical substance for neuron humor to adjust the body's development and function. Various hormones maintain a dynamic equilibrium according to the law of the unity of opposites. In the case of endocrine dyscrasia caused by diseases or some reasons, hormonal imbalance leads to some hormones' sustained action on sensitive tissues. This kind of abnormal chronic irritation may cause cell hyperplasia and canceration. Hormones with carcinogenic action refer to these that can promote histiocytes growth, such as estrogen of ovary, gonadotropic hormone of pituitary, thyrotrophic hormone and galactin, etc. To give the example of breast cancer, when lacking of pituitary and ovarian hormone promoting the growth of mammary gland, mammary gland will not grow. Undeveloped mammary tissue is hard to produce tumor. Therefore, hormone is a necessary factor to induce breast cancer. Experimental studies show that hormonal imbalance can induce tumors in thyroid gland, adenohypophysis, ovary, testicle, and adrenal cortex as well as accessory organs of uterine body, uterine neck, vagina and mammary gland. Hormone takes a long time to induce tumor; and the induction often needs a certain genetic background and environmental factors to be pathogenic conditions. Furthermore, hormone can also cooperate with other carcinogenic factors to cause canceration or act as the pathogenic condition of other factors. Some hormones, such as prostatic hormone, can promote cell differentiation and strengthen immune response. Whether the hyposecretion of prostatic hormone has an effect on canceration still needs a further study.

(4). Mycotoxin and cancer research group

For some tumors that are known to be closely related to mycotoxins, it should further study its carcinogenic factors and it should study the corresponding treatment measures in treatment and the preventive measures should be studied in anti-cancer and anti-cancer and further research should be conducted on relevant knowledge.

There are many metabolites of mold in nature, which can cause toxicity to the nervous, digestive, urinary, and blood systems of animals, **_called mycotoxin_**. There have been many reports of mycotoxin-induced acute poisoning in humans. In the past 10 years, some mycotoxins have been observed to cause carcinogenic or cancer-promoting effects on animals. Therefore, the medical community is paying more and more attention to research the mold and the relationship between mold and its toxins and human tumors.

Experimental carcinogenic mycotoxins

There have been many types of carcinogenic mycotoxins found in experimental studies. It was first discovered that **ergot fed rats** can induce neurofibroma of the ear. At first feeding rates with **ergot-infected grain** can induce the neurofibroma of ear. Then the mouldy yellowed rice polluted by Penicillium islandicum Sopp are found in Japan; and the toxin extracted from rice can cause the hepatic cirrhosis, hepatic tumor and hepatic cancer of mice and rats. Until 1960, peanut powder contaminated with Aapergillus fiavus Liak in the United Kingdom killed 100,000 turkeys. And then it was discovered that aflatoxin was carcinogenic to animals before it attracted widespread attention or Only until 1960 when one hundred thousand turkeys were poisoned to death by groundnut flour polluted by **Aspergillus flavus Liak** in England and then Aflatoxin was found to have carcinogenic action on animals, cancerogenic problem of mycotoxin finally attracted wild attention. Repeated studies prove that Aspergillus flavus Liak and its derivatives have more than ten kinds, among which the best one with carcinogenic action is B_1. Mouldy grains polluted by Aflatoxin in a liver cancer-prone area of China are mixed in feed to feed rats. After six moths, the inducing rate of liver cancer is up to 80%, which also proves the carcinogenic action of mycotoxins. This kind of feed can also cause monkeys' liver cirrhosis as well as other hepatic lesions and induce liver cancer. *Most of the induced liver cancers are hepatocellular cancers.* Furthermore, this kind of feed can lead to the adenocarcinoma of kidney, stomach and colon; intratracheal instillation can cause squamous cell carcinoma of lung; subcutaneous injection can cause local sarcoma. There are relevant reports about causing tumors in other regions, such as lachrymal gland, mammary gland and ovary. *Therefore, making a good job of mould proofing and ridding of oil and foodstuffs is important for exploring the prevention of some tumors and ensuring popular physical fitness.*

In the esophageal cancer-prone area of China, Geotrichum candidum Link abstracted from edible pickled vegetable is proved to have the cancer-promoting action. Use 0.5ml fungus medium and 0.25mg / (kg · d) methyl benzyl nitrosamine to feed a series of A mice. During two to seven months, the incidence rate of proliferative lesion, papilloma and cancer in anterior stomach of A mice is obviously higher than that of other mice only fed with nitrosamine. Use the culture of Geotrichum candidum Link to feed rats for twenty months, and then papilloma in anterior stomach is induced. Some moldy food can cause precancerous lesion and early cancer in esophageal epithelium of animals. *Some fungi abstracted from moldy food can increase the content of nitrite and secondary amine or produce nitrosamine in food. The above experiments expand the research field of the relation between fungus and tumor and also provide new clues for tumor pathogenesis.*

So far some fungi and their toxins related to tumor generation have ***both carcinogenic action and cancer-promoting action.*** This kind of dualism deserves attention.

Victory over cancer, where is the road?

XU ZE believes that the road is in scientific research - the road is in the scientific research on the prevention and treatment of cancer, and the road is researched and developed under the guidance of the scientific development concept. Through scientific research, human beings will surely overcome cancer, and will eventually overcome cancer.

Why is the road in scientific research? It is because it is necessary to know the current status of the oncology discipline, what are the problems? How to do? "Oncology" is a backward discipline in various medical sciences. Why? Because the etiology, pathogenesis, pathophysiology of oncology are not well understood.

Oncology for scientific research is still a scientific virgin land and a lot of basic scientific research is waiting.

Therefore, basic and clinical scientific research is necessary.

How to conduct scientific research on cancer?

1. What is science?

Science - is the endless of the world. Our scientific research work has always followed the scientific development concept, based on known medicine, future-oriented medicine, future-oriented science, emerging disciplines, marginal disciplines, interdisciplinary subjects, based on known science, known knowledge, to explore unknown science, Unknown knowledge. Looking forward, after calming down, working hard for a long time, practicing the scientific concept of development, and trekking on the road of scientific research, one step at a time, one step at a scientific research footprint, facing the frontiers of science, striving for innovation and progress, and adding to the research and development of cancer.

2. *What is research?*

Research is to explore the truth, nature, and law of things. Medical science research has theoretical research and clinical research. The clinical research work of our special department of Dawning Cancer Research Institute follows the following scientific research routes:

(a)   Find problems from clinical work → Ask questions → Study questions through experiments → Solve problems through clinical validation, and then solve problems for clinical problems or explain problems.

(b)   Our research is from clinical → experimental → clinical → re-experiment → re-clinical, then go back to the clinic to solve the problem.

(c)   Our research is closely combined with theory and practice. Our research topics are all from the clinical, to find the focus of clinical problems and clinical breakthroughs, after experimental research and clinical verification, and then applied to the clinic to solve Clinical practical problems. Our research follows evidence-based medicine, seeking truth from facts, speaking with facts, using data to demonstrate, measurable experimental research and clinical, validated data.

3. What is the study?

The object or target of the study is cancer. It is necessary to study how to recognize cancer. It is necessary to study how cancer is treated and treated.

To study:

1   Exploring the truth, nature, and laws of cancer;

2   the cause and development of cancer, the pathogenesis;

3   biological characteristics and biological behavior of cancer cells;

4   multi-step, multi-stage of cancer cell metastasis;

5   The relationship between cancer cells and the host, who determines the fate of cancer patients;

6   Find new ways to prevent and cure cancer. This refers to the whole process of cancer occurrence, development, metastasis, recurrence and subsequent prevention and treatment.

The whole process of cancer occurrence and development is:

Susceptibility stage → precancerous stage → early → intermediate → late stage, ie invasive stage and late stage of transfer so cancer metastasis is not the whole of cancer but only a stage of cancer.

My second book is "New Concepts and New Methods for Cancer Metastasis Treatment"; the third monograph is different for "New Concepts and New Methods for Cancer Treatment". The former is devoted to the invasion stage of cancer and cancer metastasis treatment. Cancer metastasis is only one stage of cancer development - the invasion stage, the latter is the whole process of cancer development and the prevention and treatment of the whole process. Only the whole process of prevention and treatment can overcome cancer.

4. How to study:

I have been doing oncology surgery for more than 60 years. The more patients are treated, the more patients come. I am deeply aware of:

Cancer must not only pay attention to treatment, but also pay attention to prevention in order to stop at the source. The way-out of the treatment of cancer is in the "three early days" (early detection, early diagnosis, early treatment). The way to fight cancer is prevention. More than 90% of cancers are caused by environmental factors, and protecting and restoring a good environment is an important part of preventing cancer.

Prevention cancer and cancer control and conquer cancer, why do I mention "control cancer"?

Because energy saving and pollution prevention and pollution control can effectively control the occurrence of cancer.

For prevention of cancer and cancer control, Class I prevention, Class II prevention, and Class III prevention should be used.

The current emission reduction and prevention pollution is actually Level I prevention.

Energy saving and Emission reduction and prevention pollution and Pollution reduction are scientific development and it is also a great pioneering effort to prevent cancer and control cancer for benefiting the country and people.

Research must expand its field of view, looking forward, facing the science of the future. Scientific research is mainly to study unknown new scientific knowledge, facing the future of science. Let science continue to move forward. All scientific research must advance under the guidance of the scientific development concept. Under the guidance of the scientific development concept, we should update our thinking, change our concepts, advance in reform, and be brave in innovation. Innovation must challenge traditional concepts. Cancer is a human disaster. Prevention cancer and anti-cancer are human cancer.

XU ZE thinks that victory over cancer, where is the road?

The road is in scientific research - the road is in the scientific research on the prevention and treatment of cancer, and the road is to research under the guidance of the scientific development concept.

Science - is the endless of the world, our scientific research is based on known medicine, facing future medicine and emerging disciplines and marginal disciplines and interdisciplinary subjects and is based on known science to explore future science and unknown knowledge. Looking forward, after calming down and working hard for a long time, on the scientific road, we have to travel hard, step by step, and to face the frontier of science, strive for innovation and progress, to add bricks and tiles to the research halls for conquering cancer.

Prevention of cancer and anti-cancer

Conquer cancer and launch the general attack to cancer

Condense wisdom and conquer cancer

Conquer cancer and Launch a general attack

Multidisciplinary to overcome cancer and launch the general attack of cancer and the research base of the Cancer Research Group - Science City

General Design, Blueprint and Preparation Work (2) (Volume 2)

Conquer cancer and launch a total attack

"The multidisciplinary of overcoming cancer and launching a total attack and the scientific research base of cancer research group – the Science City"

The total design and the blueprint and the preparatory work (2)

(Volume II)

TABLE OF CONTENTS

Volume II

FOREWORD

This book is used to conquer cancer and to launch the general attack on cancer and to create the Science City for conquering cancer. *XZ-C's overall design, planning, and blueprint of the scientific research projects for conquering cancer is the scientific thinking and theoretical innovation and experimental basis for conquering cancer.* It is the overall strategic reform and development of cancer treatment in China. It is **my 60 years of experience in medical work** and **30 years of scientific research results** and **the scientific and technological innovation and the scientific thinking and scientific research wisdom** which conquering cancer is as the research direction. Now It is planned to set up a test area in the Huangjiahu University City of Wuhan City. The research project will be implemented by experts and professors of the research team.

The research plan of conquering overcome cancer is a key scientific research in the world and a frontier of science.

On January 12, 2016, US President Barack Obama proposed the National Cancer Program "Conquering Cancer" in his State of the Union address, and named the Cancer Moon Shot, which was implemented by Vice President Biden. The specific plan is unknown.

Cancer is a disaster for all mankind. It must fight globally. The people of the world should work together to gather wisdom and to advance together to overcome cancer.

The disaster of cancer covers the whole world. People all over the world are eager to hope to overcome cancer one day. It is hoped that the state, government, experts, scholars and scientists can find out anti-cancer measures to keep people away from cancer.

XZ-C proposed the research program of conquering cancer and launching the total attack

The overall strategic reform and development of cancer treatment

Professor Xu Ze (XU ZE), Honorary President of Wuhan Anti-Cancer Research Association, proposed the following 4 items of the feasibility report and the total design of the research plan for conquering cancer and launching the general attack of cancer in July 2015

(1) For the first time in the international community it is put forward :

"The necessity and the feasibility of the report to capture the total attack of cancer"

- ----The overall strategy of cancer strategy is changed from focusing on treatment into focusing on prevention and treatment at the equal attention.

(2) for the first time in the international community it was put forward :

"To build the prevention and treatment hospitals during the whole process of cancer development and occurrence"

(Global demonstration of the hospital with prevention and treatment of cancer)

"the imagination and feasibility report of building the hospital with the prevention and treatment of cancer during the whole anti-cancer process"

-------*Describe the necessity and feasibility of establishing a complete prevention and treatment hospital*

(3) <u>*For the first time in the international community it was put forward :*</u>

<u>*"To build the basic design and feasibility report of a total attack to capture cancer and science city"*</u>

------ *is equivalent to design the whole framework about design with Chinese charasterics of conquering cancer.*

(4) <u>*For the first time in the international community it is put forward :*</u>

<u>*"In building a moderately society at the same time, the proposed" ride research "- for the medical science research of cancer prevention and cancer control and the necessity and feasibility report of cancer prevention and treatment"*</u>

- Adhere to the Chinese characteristics of control cancer and cancer prevention path

These four international research projects are the first time to be put forward in the international, are the international initiative, the international leader, open up a new field of anti-cancer research.

Change from paying attention to the heavy treatment and light prevention into paying equal attention to both cancer prevention and treatment in an attempt to achieve lower incidence of cancer and improve cancer cure rate.

Opening up new areas of research is possible to conquer cancer, even conquering cancer. It is b<u>*ecause for a century people have been based on cancer treatment, and the treatment is based on killing cancer cells*</u>.

However, chemotherapeutic drugs are first-order kinetics, and it is impossible to kill cancer cells completely. The time for patients to effectively kill cancer cells by chemotherapy is only 3-5 days of intravenous drip, which has the effect of killing cancer cells. After that, there is no effect of killing cancer cells. It is only a short time to kill (3-5 days), not once and for all; after 3-5 days, the cancer cells continue to divide and proliferate, so it can only be relieved for a short time and it cannot be cured and can only kill a certain number of cancer cells, and there will still be cancer cells constantly produced. Therefore, its efficacy is defined as "alleviation", and the remission time is only 4 weeks or more, and it will still recur and metastasize. Therefore, chemotherapy cannot cure cancer, and cannot rely on chemotherapy to overcome cancer. Although it has been used for more than half a century, cancer is still the leading cause of death for both urban and rural residents.

__This research project, which was first proposed by the Chinese at the international level, can benefit mankind and revitalize China and shock the world. It needs courage and needs wisdom and strength and needs a scientific basis to propose to overcome cancer and to launch the general attack on cancer.__

This research project was first proposed by Professor Xu Ze for the feasibility report and application for the first time in the world. Under the leadership of the province and the city, the Wuhan Anticancer Research Association will undertake and implementing and carrying out XZ-C's Basic assumptions and design of conquering cancer and launching the general attack of cancer

The first scientific research program is proposed a feasibility report and apply for the preparation by Professor Xu Ze in the international community for the first time. It will be conducted by the Wuhan anti-cancer research under the leadership of the provincial and municipal leaders.

The implementation of the "XZ-C attack on cancer to start the basic idea and design":

(Xu ZE) Professor proposed to overcome the cancer and to launch the general offensive ideas, strategies, planning sketches, and proposed the total design, guidance of the Science City of overcoming the cancer to launch a total attack, commanded "to build a science city which have the medical, teaching, research and development of conquering cancer and launch the total attack". First of all, to build " the hospital of the prevention and treatment of cancer during the whole process of cancer occurrence and development --- - the global demonstration of the cancer prevention and treatment hospital."

The purpose is:

① *reduce the incidence of cancer*

② *improve cancer cure rate*

③ *extend the survival period*

④ *improve the quality of life*

⑤ *reduce complications*

二

It was proposed to establish the test area of conquering cancer work group (station) in the province or city

Professor Xu Ze proposed the overall design and planning and blueprint to conquer cancer and to launch the total attack

To set up the following groups:

1). *The academic Committee to overcome the Cancer*

2). *The building work group of the Science City (the science city of conquering cancer and launching a total attack with the medical, teaching, research and development science school)*

1. To set up the Academic Committee of overcoming cancer

The conditions of the academic members:

Have the genuine talent or skills and have the academic achievement on the basic research or clinical work of cancer and have academic results and have monograph, editor, patent, thesis and practical clinical experience and have experimental research results and its research and academics is taking the research direction as capturing cancer and have the leading talent of leadership and organization of conquering cancer. It must have both ability and the moral.

Academic committee

Consultant:

(Leading scientists who have academic achievements in cancer research)

Chairman:

Vice Chairman: 17 well-known experts, professors, academic leaders or leading scientists

Members: 36 are academic leaders, experts and professors

2. The building working group of the Science City (the science city with the medical, teaching, research and development to attack the cancer and to launch a total attack)

The building division of labor of the "Science City" with capturing the cancer as the research direction and the main task :

1). *The financing group: (financing, investment)*

2). *The building group: (site, house, decoration, equipment)*

3). *The academic group: (content: multidisciplinary subject set, multi-disciplinary research group set, compulsory courses and elective courses set, according to medical, teaching, research, hair were implemented, the laboratory set up and established)*

4). *The preparation of the Secretariat Office: Team leader:*

3. The working group with research results, transformation and development of the province of attacking the cancer and launching a total offensive

Leading group

Leader:

Deputy head:

Co-leader:

Department of Education:

Science and Technology Department:

Health Commission:

Environmental Protection Agency:

Transformation, development office:

Secretariat:

XZ-C proposed to conquer cancer and launch a total attack to cancer, that is, prevention cancer, cancer control, cancer treatment three fleets go hand in hand; prevention and treatment are at the equal attention, so the they are both involved:

① **Education department**: to cultivate the general offensive multidisciplinary senior personnel, the establishment of innovative tumor medical college and tumor multidisciplinary senior personnel training courses, teaching and research group (teaching and research) should have a better laboratory or laboratory.

② **Science and technology departments**: to carry out the "three early" research, research early diagnosis of new reagents, new technologies, new methods, open up new areas of anti-cancer research, new technologies, new methods, new industries, eyes forward, Three early ".

③ **Health and Social Health Department**: cancer treatment, anti-cancer, cancer is the management of the work of the health sector, should be anti-governance and both.

④ **environmental protection departments**: should open up new areas of environmental protection and anti-cancer research, new technologies, new industries, because 80% of cancer and the environment is closely related. Should be from the clothing, food, live, anti-cancer, from the environment, small environmental anti-cancer, first monitoring, qualitative, quantitative, set the standard, the establishment of multi-project laboratory, macro, micro, ultra-microscopic research, Methods and measures.

4. The test area of the province or city to attack cancer work group (station)

the setting up working group of the "Science City"

the chief architect, president, chairman of the General Academic Committee is for Professor Xu Ze.

The preparatory group of the "Science City" to build scientific research program:

① *innovative full-scale anti-cure hospital - are all disciplines and professors, each preparatory group has 12 professors, experts*

② *innovative tumor medical school - are all disciplines and professors, each preparatory group has 12 professors, experts*

③ *Innovative Cancer Research Institute - are professors and professors, each preparatory group has 12 professors, experts*

④ *experimental medical cancer animal experimental center - are all disciplines and professors, each preparatory group has 12 professors, experts*

⑤ *innovative nano-pharmaceutical companies - all disciplines and professors, each preparatory group has 12 professors, experts*

5. Anti-Cancer Research Association and Shuguang Hing Conversion Medical Center

The working group of XZ-C research results transformation and development

(1) transformation of medicine, research and development working group:

Honorary leader:

Leader:

Deputy head:

Co-leader:

Director of the Centre:

Center Secretary-General:

Deputy Secretary-General:

(2) Purpose:

(3) Method:

The Establishment of the Scientific Research Base of conquering cancer and launching the total attack of cancer---- the Science City

The total design and blueprint of "The research base of conquering cancer and launching the total offensive - Science City"

The total design and preparation work of "Science City"

(A) how to overcome cancer? XZ-C provided:

"Conquer Cancer and Launch the Total Attack"

1. Why is it put forward to overcome cancer? Look at the present situation:

(1) The status quo of the incidence of cancer is : the more treatment and the more patients

Today the incidence of cancer in China is 3.12 million new cases of cancer per year, and an average of 8550 new cancer patients per day. Six people were diagnosed with cancer every minute in the country.

(2) the status of cancer mortality is high and has been the first cause of death in urban and rural areas in China

Today China's cancer mortality rate is 2.7 million deaths per year due to cancer deaths, an average of 7,500 people died of cancer every day, every 7 dead people that one died of cancer.

Cancer in China is so high incidence, the more the rule of the patient, the high mortality rate, should be a major issue of national economy and people's livelihood, should be a major issue of people's health, should be the people's major suffering and disaster.

Human beings should not sit still, physicians should not do nothing, leadership should not do nothing, I think we should put forward "to overcome cancer." "Declaring war on cancer" is the time, should gather wisdom, overcome cancer.

2. Why did Professor Xu Ze propose to overcome cancer and to launch a total attack? Look at the current status of cancer treatment:

(1) the current status of cancer treatment:

Although the application of the traditional three treatment for nearly a hundred years, tens of thousands of cancer patients to bear the release, chemotherapy, but the results? So far the cancer is still the first cause of death, although the patients are carried out a formal, systematic radiotherapy or chemotherapy, or radiotherapy + chemotherapy, it still failed to prevent cancer metastasis and recurrence, little effect.

(2) the status quo of the mode of the current tumor hospital or the oncology

(1) go all out to focus on treatment, for the middle and late cancer, depleted human and financial resources, and failed to achieve lower mortality, prolong survival, reduce morbidity, cancer is still the first cause of death in urban and rural areas.

(2) only treatment, or paying more attention to heavy treatment and less attention to prevention or defense, the more treatment and the more patients.

(3) ignored the "three early", ignoring the prevention.

(4) many large hospitals, university hospitals have not established a laboratory, can not carry out the basic research of cancer or clinical basic research, because if no basic research breakthrough, the clinical efficacy is difficult to improve. "Oncology" is still a backward discipline in all medical disciplines today. why? It is because the etiology, pathogenesis, and pathophysiology of "oncology" are not well understood. People still lack sufficient understanding of the mechanism of its pathogenesis and cancer cell metastasis. Therefore, the current cancer treatment plan is still quite blind, so it is necessary to establish a laboratory for basic research and clinical basic research.

The status quo is:

a. through a century road, the hospital model is: heavy treatment and light prevention or defense, or only treatment, the result is: the more treatment and the more patients.

b. through a century road, the treatment model is: to aim at the late invasion and metastasis of the advanced patients and it exhausted human and financial resources ; the result is that the mortality rate is high.

How to do? It should change the current treatment mode and the hospital mode, and it is put forward to overcome cancer and to launch the total attack.

3. what is the total attack of conquering cancer?

XZ-C proposed to the general idea and design of capturing cancer.

The total attack is to conduct the work in full swing, simultaneously for the three stages such as cancer prevention, control and treatment during the whole process of cancer development and occurrence.

That is:

Prevention of cancer - before the formation of cancer

Cancer control - malignant transformation of precancerous lesions

Cancer treatment - has formed a foci or metastases

The Objective: To reduce the incidence of cancer, reduce cancer mortality, improve the cure rate, prolong survival, improve the quality of life, reduce complications.

The total design and the blueprint and the preparatory work of " the research base to conquer cancer and to launch the total attack – the Science City"

XZ-C (XU ZE - China) proposed:

How to overcome cancer by I see one:

1. **How to overcome cancer? To overcome cancer, it must create "the innovative molecular cancer medical school"**

---- in order to overcome cancer it is built "the science city of conquering cancer and launching the total attack of cancer" by one

(1) Why is it to create "innovative molecular cancer medical school"?

Because: (1) the current status of cancer scholars are mainly the radiotherapy and chemotherapy talent; however, in order to conquer cancer and launch a total attack, it needs the multi-disciplinary talents.

① **to overcome cancer, the talent is the key.** It is to train the relevant personnel who can participate in the capture of cancer, launch the total attack. The talent must be genuine talent and have the technology *and theory and must both ability and political integrity and medicine is benevolence, the moral is the first.*

Personnel must have knowledge of undergraduate knowledge, life science knowledge, knowledge of Chinese medicine, molecular biology, genetic engineering, environmental science, environmental science, medical multidisciplinary knowledge, immunology, virology, endocrinology, immunopharmacology and so on.

② **to overcome cancer, talent is the key, how to train talent is the key.** Research of cancer talent requires a number of disciplinary knowledge and technology, to genetic engineering, molecular biology immunology, virological experimental personnel, knowledge must also have technology, hands-on ability, technology needs knowledge, so that under the guidance of the theory, The development of high-end technology, the need to tackle the first-class talent, we must concentrate on, calm down, concentrate on this work. Where does talent come from? It is based on their own training and that they create their own machine to hatch the talent.

③ **to overcome the cancer, start the total attack and move forward together with the prevention of the cancer + control cancer + the treatment of the cancer and the three are together, so the teaching plan must develop cancer prevention science talent, the cancer disease control personnel and the teaching content and knowledge and the course related anti-cancer and preventive medicine.**

At present, anti-cancer, cancer control talent is scarce, urgent need to accelerate training to meet the urgent need to launch a general attack.

In view of more than 90% of the cancer caused by environmental factors or closely related to the current we are ongoing energy-saving emission reduction, sewage pollution control, this policy and work and anti-cancer, cancer control work has a great relevance, Related talent.

④ the current educational content can not keep up with the development of the times. **To overcome the cancer it must develop the modern high-tech disciplines and it must have a good laboratory, but in the current it lacks of the laboratory talent. For attacking the cancer and launching a total attack and anti-cancer and controlling cancer, it is lacking of the laboratory experimental modern high-tech talent and the intermediate specialist talent who can go deep into the community to prevent cancer, cancer control capacity.**

It should strengthen the establishment of laboratory personnel for the tertiary institutions. Modern life science and technology progress rapidly and the genetic engineering and the molecular biology and the cell inheritance rapid develop.

Because Professor Xu Ze (XZ) proposed to attack the cancer and launch a general attack, which is unprecedented in human work, must develop the high-tech talent and technology with the basic medicine, clinical medicine, life sciences, Chinese and Western medicine, preventive medicine, experimental medicine, molecular level skills and it must personally practice, create experience, develop medicine. Therefore, at the same time it is to establish the graduate school, to cultivate thesenior scientific and technological personnel for attacking the cancer .

(2) how to set up "innovative molecular level cancer medical school"?

1) to overcome cancer, talent is the key, how to train talent is the key? People who study cancer must require multidisciplinary talent and technology. The current world countries are concentrated on a large number of scientific research elite research, therefore, the education sector to accelerate the development of anti-cancer research multidisciplinary senior personnel services.

We build "innovative molecular cancer medical school" which is to attack the cancer and launch a total offensive training research personnel training services. Professor Xu Ze proposed to attack the cancer launched a general attack, is unprecedented in human work, must create their own experience, must practice in person, this is a new cement road, every step will leave the eternal scientific footprints, so I suggest a Department of Education Department of the Office of the Department of Cancer Medical College of the leadership, to create experience.

2) the current global and China's oncology is the main treatment of talent, and attack the cancer launched a total attack, compared to cancer + cancer + cancer (anti-+ control) to carry out simultaneously, troika, go hand in hand, you need Prevention of talent, prevention of scientific talents, public health department of talent, prevention of medical college talent, urgent need to prevent and control talent.

3) the current cancer treatment of the object is mainly invasive, middle or late transfer or recurrence of the patient, the main treatment for the traditional three treatment, surgery, radiotherapy and chemotherapy, and attack the

cancer to attack the total attack was anti + + control, Focus on the left shift, the main attack of the object is mainly "three early", early in situ cancer, precancerous lesions, "three early" diagnosis and treatment technology. Early can only qualitative, and some can not locate, it only needs a small surgery, generally it does not need the big surgery and the early cancer prognosis is good and can be complete cured and "three early" in situ cancer, precancerous lesions, severe atypical hyperplasia do not have to put Chemotherapy.

4) how to overcome cancer? Training talent is the key.

How to train talent? How to cultivate modern high-tech talent, to attack the cancer launched a total attack, the goal catch up with the international advanced level, to obtain the original innovation, the leading international level of scientific and technological achievements, the key is the educational institutions, the teaching and research group should have a good laboratory to cultivate cancer HiTech Personnel.

Because the innovative molecular cancer medical school teaching content includes: modern medical science knowledge and technology, life science knowledge and technology, modern biomedical knowledge and technology, traditional Chinese medicine knowledge, experimental medicine knowledge and technology **... ... these modern science is the developing science. Science - is the endless frontier, the rapid development of modern high-tech, with each passing day, the quality of university teachers and teaching quality must also keep up with modern high-tech development, advancing with the times.**

University teachers should have a dual task on the shoulders, one is to improve teaching, the second is the development of science.

University teachers should have a good laboratory for scientific research, based on the known science, to explore the unknown science, for the future science, emerging disciplines, marginal disciplines, interdisciplinary, scientific frontier, for innovation and development.

To conquer cancer must have the talents with multiple skills with the following skills: immune and caner; virus and cancer; endocrine hormones and cancer; fungi and cancer; molecular biology and cancer; genes and cancer; environment and the relationship between cancer and cancer; Cancer; traditional Chinese medicine and cancer; chronic inflammation and cancer.

It is necessary to cultivate high-level professionals with the prevention of control and cancer control and treatment of cancer . Education is the backing of cancer. The education must cultivate talents for the purpose of attacking cancer, and the people must have this professional theoretical knowledge and professional skills., Talent must both ability and political integrity, medicine is benevolence, legislation for the first.

(3) **how to run an innovative molecular cancer medical school in order to train the personnel for attacking the cancer and launching a total offensive? It should build a good laboratory.**

It is necessary to have a good laboratory, to carry out scientific research, to be based on known science, to explore unknown science, and to face emerging science in the future.

China's universities and Europe and the United States compared to the gap between the size of the school and the number of teachers and students, the main gap is the lack of high-tech laboratories, the US technology boom, high-tech development, Attention to science and technology experiments, attention to the laboratory. Each year, a large number of international students, visiting scholars to study in the United States, are basically in the laboratory work and study. China University and the United States and Britain and other countries of the University of the main gap lies in the United States and Britain and other universities modern high-tech laboratory everywhere, excellent equipment, teaching and research group of basic teaching work in the laboratory, research, research, training graduate students, students to teach students to innovation, To develop new areas of research, a talent, a master.

Massachusetts Institute of Technology, the scale is small, the number of teachers and students only a few thousand people, but the school had 38 Nobel Prize winners, won a total of 39 Nobel Prize in Science, one of them won two Connaught Award. Ranking the highest in the world famous universities. Because the school has many modern high-tech high-level laboratories, laboratory talent, there are many academic masters, pioneered a number of cutting-edge research areas, strict style of study, rigorous and rigorous.

This shows that the laboratory is the incubation of scientific research results, the laboratory is the training of personnel incubator.

University professors should not only talk about the knowledge of the textbooks, but also should talk about today's new progress, the development of new trends,

new achievements and unknown knowledge, a mentor should have a good laboratory, it is possible to guide graduate students to conduct scientific research, Papers, development science.

To have the Development of science, scientific and technological innovation, the laboratory is the key condition.

It should vigorously build laboratories and train more the high-tech talent and have more innovative results.

(1) training talent is two ways

① founder of Cancer Medical School

② founder of Cancer Graduate School

(2) Method:

① to overcome the cancer to mobilize the total attack academic committee members and Wuhan anti-cancer research professor and interested in conception of cancer professor, 100 professors, mentor with 100 graduate students and Master and Ph. D students.

② Graduate School is teaching, experiment, practice (morning clinical, surgery, outpatient, afternoon into the laboratory

To Guide academic thinking, scientific research ethics, experimental methods, scientific research

③ academic committee professor according to the clinical problems must solve the clinical basis of the problem ... ... and so out of 100 topics, postgraduate academic committee to discuss the subject to decide to get the Master and Ph.D students.

50 master questions - must be a result, to solve practical problems, clinical can be practical, the patient benefit

50 doctoral thesis - heavy experiment, heavy practice, heavy technology, heavy theory, re-scientific thinking, heavy theoretical basis, must be a result, innovative thinking, or a patent, clinical application value, achievements, results, patents, papers, Must be innovative, we must pay attention to scientific research ethics.

Medical is benevolence, legislation for the first

Master and Ph.D students must have both ability and political integrity.

(3) Graduate School and the Provincial Natural Science Foundation, Science and Technology Department, Association for collaboration

(4) within three years it must product 100 research papers or achievements, or patents, or Chinese herbal anti-cancer new drugs, focusing on "three early" new reagents, new technologies, new methods, new drugs.

The new drugs, new methods, new technologies, new concepts, new theories, Chinese and Western medications for anti - cancer metastasis and anti-cancer recurrence and the prevention of cancer

(2) how to set up "innovative molecular cancer medical school"? How to implement and create? It should apply for provincial education department leadership and support.

五.

XZ-C puts forward how to conquer cancer by I see two:

2. How to conquer cancer? In order to conquer cancer, the Innovative Molecular Oncology Institute must be created

------- In order to overcome cancer, "the science city of conquering cancer and launching the total attack of cancer " is set up by one

(1) Why should we found the "the Innovative Molecular Oncology Institute"?

Because:

1. "Oncology" is still the current medical science in the most backward of a discipline. Why? It is because the etiology and pathogenesis and pathophysiology of the "oncology" are not yet clear, there are a lot of basic theoretical problems yet not to understand clearly on the biological characteristics of cancer cells; the molecular mechanism of cancer cell metastasis is still lack of understanding; it is involving in the virus, immune, fungal, endocrine hormones, the environment and other carcinogenic factors; it must have the multidisciplinary research.

The study of oncology is the most complex subject in medical research. It involves multidisciplinary knowledge and theory. It is necessary to set up a specialist group closely related to cancer to conduct an in-depth study in order to help overcome the total attack of cancer.

2. Therefore, the creation of "Innovative Molecular Cancer Institute" is to conquer cancer and to launch a total attack for the exploration of cancer etiology, pathogenesis, cancer cell metastasis mechanism, immune mechanism, to perform in-depth study and for the organization of further study of science closely related to cancer . It is based on the knowledge and theory of this discipline and known medicine to explore the subject of unknown knowledge, future medicine, edge disciplines, interdisciplinary, and to understand the causes and mechanisms of cancer, so as to provide effective intervention for cancer prevention and treatment measures in order to help overcoming cancer.

(2) Why should we build a cancer research institute?

Because:

In order to overcome the cancer, we must build "innovative molecular tumor research institute" closely combined with clinical practice, cancer research.

To overcome cancer, where is the road?

I believe that the road is in the scientific research, the road is on the scientific research of the prevention and treatment of cancer, the road is to explore the experimental basic research cause and pathogenesis and pathophysiology of cancer, the road is in the scientific research of the whole process of occurrence and development, the road is in the reform and development for the traditional therapy, the road is in the multi-disciplinary research, the road is in the study of the prevention and treatment of cancer metastasis and recurrence, the road is in the "three early" study.

Through the scientific research of cancer prevention and treatment, mankind will overcome cancer, and ultimately will overcome cancer.

1). How to conquer cancer I see one:

The road of scientific research is to explore the cause of cancer, pathogenesis, pathophysiology of experimental basic research.

The author believes that the development of cancer research is an urgent need for the current status of oncology. It is important to recognize the problems in the current status of the oncology discipline. What should I do?

Although cancer treatment has been going on for more than a century, it has entered the second decade of the 21st century, but "oncology" is still the most backward discipline in the current medical sciences. Why? It is because the etiology, pathogenesis, and pathophysiology of "oncology" are not well understood. Oncology is still a scientific virgin for scientific research, and it needs a lot of basic scientific research and clinical basic research.

Although the traditional three major treatment methods (surgery, radiotherapy, chemotherapy) have been applied for nearly a hundred years, thousands of cancer patients have undergone radiotherapy and chemotherapy. But what is the result?

So far, the rate of cancer mortality is still the first cause of death for urban and rural residents in China. How should the road go? It should be deeply introspected, in-depth analysis, and in-depth study.

Why is this so? The main reasons are the following:

1. *The cause of cancer is still not clear, the pathogenesis is still not clear, the pathophysiology is still not clear, and there are a large number of basic theoretical issues that have not been clearly understood.*

2. *There is still insufficient understanding of the biological characteristics and biological behavior of cancer cells.*

3. *There is still insufficient understanding of the molecular mechanism of cancer cell metastasis.*

2). How to overcome cancer? I see two:

The road of the scientific research lies in the development of multidisciplinary research, the formation of relevant specialist groups, and specializing in-depth basic and clinical research.

Anti-cancer research needs to involve multiple disciplines, not only clinical medicine, but also the participation of many interdisciplinary, interdisciplinary, and basic disciplines. Cancer metastasis and recurrence studies include internal medicine, surgery, radiation, endocrine, drugs, immunity, molecular biology, viruses, biological information, genetic engineering, life sciences, molecular chemistry, enzyme chemistry, environmental protection, traditional Chinese medicine, and laboratory. Our city has the above-mentioned talents in various disciplines and has a certain foundation. We can organize all parties' scientific and technological strengths, work together, and take the road of scientific research and cooperation to jointly improve the level of anti-cancer metastasis and recurrence, and benefit the millions of cancer patients.

3). The following specialist groups closely related to cancer should be established, specializing in basic and clinical research.

In view of the multidisciplinary knowledge and theory of oncology research, it is necessary to form relevant specialist groups to further study.

Based on the known knowledge and known medicine of the discipline, to study and explore the unknown knowledge, future medicine, marginal disciplines and interdisciplinary subjects of the discipline, in order to help overcome cancer, the following specialist groups should be established. In the future, it is possible to form new disciplines or interdisciplinary and new industries.

(1) Immunization and Cancer Research Group: Laboratory;

(2) Virus and Cancer Research Group: Laboratory;

(3) Endocrine Hormone and Cancer Research Group: Laboratory;

(4) Mycotoxins and Cancer Research Group: Laboratory;

(5) Environmental and Cancer Research Group: Laboratory;

(6) ....;

(7) ....;

(8) ....;

In order to conquer cancer, we must establish the Institute of Innovative Molecular Oncology.

First, establish a multidisciplinary and cancer research group to study the new reagents, new technologies and new methods of "three early" to improve the diagnosis and treatment of "three early".

At present, CT, MRI and other diagnostic methods are very advanced, and the hardware is very good, but once diagnosed, it is in the middle and late stage, and should try to study the early diagnosis method and the early treatment method and the early diagnosis method, early treatment method for precancerous lesions and precancerous conditions.

At present, most of them are morphological or influential diagnosis, all need to grow to a certain volume to be diagnosed. If you can find research from serum, immunity, etc., you may find a diagnosis like syphilis from Kahn reaction and Wassermann reaction and Typhoid from Widal test, and other early diagnosis methods.

(3) how to create "the innovative molecular tumor research"? How to implement and create?

To build an innovative molecular tumor research institute

Sixth floor	11	12
Fifth floor	9	10
Fourth floor	7	8
Third floor	5`	6
Second floor	3	4
First floor	1	2

First, rent a 6-storey building closely combining with the actual needs of the clinic; first carry out a number of multi-disciplinary and cancer-related research, and try first.

In the future, we will gradually strengthen scientific research projects and add relevant research groups.

Rent for three years and pay the rent for one year each year.

The First floor

(1) immunology and cancer research group and laboratory

(2) virus and cancer research group and laboratory

The Second floor

(3) endocrine hormone and cancer research group and laboratory

(4) Environmental and Cancer Research Group and Laboratory

The Third floor

(5) Chinese medicine and cancer research group and laboratory

(6) "three early" and cancer research group and laboratory

The Fourth floor

(7) fungi and cancer research group and laboratory

(8) Molecular Biology and Cancer Research Group and Laboratory

The Fifth floor

(9) Genetic Engineering and Cancer Research Group and Laboratory

(10) precancerous lesions and cancer research group and laboratory

Sixth floor laboratory, office

The above-mentioned building

First, a batch of scientific research projects will be carried out, which will be linked to the department of "preparing the hospital with the prevention and treatment of cancer during the whole process of the development and occurrence ."

Preparation for the "Innovative Molecular Oncology Research Institute" is to overcome the actual problems of clinical prevention, control and treatment of cancer. The study is based on clinical problems. Why is an innovative molecular tumor research institute to carry out cancer research set up? It is an urgent need of the current status of oncology, and it is necessary to recognize what problems exist in the current status of oncology, and what to do?

Although cancer treatment has been going on for more than a century and is now in its second decade of the 21ˢᵗ century, "oncology" is still the most backward discipline in the current medical sciences. Why? It is because the etiology, pathogenesis, pathophysiology of "oncology" are not well understood. The oncology discipline is still a scientific virgin for scientific research, and it needs a lot of basic scientific research and clinical basic research. Although the traditional three major treatment methods (surgery, radiotherapy, chemotherapy) have been applied for nearly a hundred years, thousands of cancer patients have undergone radiotherapy and chemotherapy. But what is the result? The cancer death rate so far is still the first cause of death in urban and rural residents of China. How should the road go? It should be deeply introspected, in-depth analysis, and in-depth study.

Therefore, it is necessary to build an innovative molecular tumor research institute, carry out basic research on cancer, anti-cancer metastasis and recurrence, and must conduct basic research on cancer-bearing animal models to study the laws and mechanisms of cancer cell metastasis, because if there is no breakthrough in basic research, The clinical efficacy is difficult to improve.

Professor Xu Ze pointed out:

The research topics and research routes are based on the following research routes:

- The study is all from clinical → experimental → clinical → re-experiment → re-clinical. Go back to the clinic to solve the problem and benefit the patient.

- The theory and practice are closely combined. The topics are all from the clinical, to find the focus of clinical problems and clinical breakthroughs, after experimental research and clinical verification, and then applied to the clinic to solve clinical practical problems.

- Evidence-based medicine, seeking truth from facts, strong scientific, using facts to speak and to demonstrate, have measurable experimental research and clinically validated data, and attach importance to the accumulation of original data.

- ***Evaluation criteria***: long live, long survival time, good quality of life, clinical observation 3 to 5 years, or even 8-10 years, can be used to initially evaluate the long-term efficacy.

Innovative Molecular Cancer Institute

The study of oncology is the most complex and difficult problem in medical research. It involves multidisciplinary knowledge and theory. It should be organized with the following special groups, which are closely related to cancer, and specialize in basic and clinical research; it should be based on the known knowledge of the discipline, known medicine, to explore the unknown knowledge of the discipline and the future of medicine and the edge disciplines and the interdisciplinary in order to help overcoming cancer. In the future it may form the new disciplines and the new industries.

Based on more than 30 years of scientific research experience, Professor Xu Ze think of that the following disciplines are related cancer occurrence and development and pathophysiology and pathogenesis and metastasis and recurrence and treatment so that it is proposed to first set up the following disciplines research groups.

The following specialized groups should be set up :

(1) Immunology and Cancer Research Group (Section):

The recent clinical research task should be (to carry out the following work)

1   *Detection and evaluation of immune function status of cancer patients.*

2   *monitoring the efficacy of immunomodulatory treatment for cancer patients.*

3   *quantitative monitoring of immune function status of patients with radiotherapy and chemotherapy.*

(2) Virus and Cancer Research Group (Department):

1   *Funding to establish a laboratory for virus and cancer culture centers and to identify professionals and academic leaders.*

2   *fundraising to establish a cancer cell culture room.*

3   *Funding to establish a laboratory for cancer animal models.*

4   *It is proposed to cooperate with Dr. Li of Yale University in the United States to conduct HPV detection.*

(3) Hormone (endocrine) and cancer research groups and laboratories

1) hormone clinical patient test

2) Clinical laboratory observation of hormone imbalance and cancer

3) application of hormones and carcinogenic problems

4) precancerous lesions and hormone observation

(4) Environmental and Cancer Research Related Groups (Department) and Laboratory

1) Investigate and control the risk factors of common malignant tumors, and enter the in-depth intervention study

2) monitoring pollution carcinogenic data and researching and developing the measures of the prevention cancer and cancer control measures

For:

(a) food, grocery;

(b) Water pollution, beverages

(c) house decoration;

(d) Air pollution, quantitative data monitoring of carcinogens in factories and automobile exhausts

3) monitoring environmental pollution carcinogenic data, research on anti-cancer measures, research and development interventions

4) emission reduction and environmental protection, and the establishment of "8+1" prevention cancer and anti-cancer alliance

5) Established prevention cancer and anti-cancer information and communication newspaper - "People's Medicine" from the big living environment, living in a small environment to prevent cancer

All of the above special study groups belong to various disciplines of the hospital and are located in hospitals.

About one year later, I will try to set up a research institute for each special discipline, and strive for the establishment of a general research institute.

The above research institutions:

Department → Research Group → Research Institute → Purpose, Task, Planning, Implementation, Coordination of Projects, Projects, and Objectives; Scientific research achievements, technological innovation.

To take the conquering cancer as the direction of cancer research, to

improve the overall level of medical care, to benefit patients.

The general design of the subject research of the above special research groups, the general manager of the discipline: Professor Xu Ze

We are preparing to build the "Innovative Molecular Oncology Research Institute" to conduct a series of multidisciplinary studies to conquer cancer and to launch the general attack on cancer. Professor Xu Ze proposed to overcome cancer and to launch the general attack of cancer, which is unprecedented in human history. It is necessary to create experience by itself and must practice it personally. Therefore, I suggest that the staff of a provincial science and technology department be the leader of the Cancer Research Institute (secretary) to create experience.

六

XZ-C proposed how to conquer cancer by I see the three:

3.How to conquer cancer? In order to conquer cancer, we must create "the innovative molecular tumor hospital" (the global demonstration of the hospital with the prevention and treatment of the whole process of the cancer occurrence and development)

-------*in order to conquer cancer, one of setting up the science city of conquering cancer and launching the total attack of cancer*

(1) Why is it to create "the hospital of the innovative molecular tumor with the prevention and treatment during the whole process of cancer occurrence and development"?

Because:

1. *the existing problems in the mode of setting up the cancer hospital in the current global and China and oncology department*

A). go all out, the focus of treatment on the advanced cancer patients with middle, late, metastatic, recurrence so that the curative effect is poor, the manpower and financial resources are exhausted, and the mortality rate is not reduced, the cure rate is increased, the morbidity rate is lowered, and the mortality rate is still the first cause of death for urban and rural residents.

B). only treatment without prevention, or pay attention to treatment with light prevention, the patient gets more and more, or attention of treatment and no prevention; the more treatment and the more patients.

2. Cancer hospital or hospital oncology department and the hospital model in the current global and in China are the treatment of hospitals; the objects of the treatment of patients are in the middle and late stages and metastatic; the effect is very poor.

The hospital models: all are the treatment hospitals and attention of treatment and light prevention or defense, or only treatment and no prevention.

The treatment model: all aim at the middle stages or late stages patients or the advanced patients with advanced cancer metastasis.

It should (must) reform:

To reform of the hospital model: *it should be changed into prevention and control and treatment at the same equal.*

To reform of treatment model: *it should be changed to focus on early, precancerous lesions … … and so on, the way out of cancer treatment is in the "three early", must study the diagnosis of the new technologies, new methods, new reagents of "three early" ; the early cancer can be cured.*

③ Therefore, to create " the hospital of the innovative molecular tumor with the prevention and treatment during the whole process of occurrence and development; " in order to overcome cancer, it should reform the hospital model and change the treatment model, XZ-C proposed to overcome cancer and launch a total attack.

What is called as conquering cancer and launching the total attack?

The total attack is to carry out in a comprehensive work of three stages of cancer prevention and cancer control and cancer treatment during the whole process of cancer occurrence and development, and synchronize, troika, go hand in hand, keep pace, reform the current hospital mode, change the current treatment model.

Namely: the reform of the current treatment-focused model. To change the current hospital model of focus on treatment in the middle and late stage; to reform treatment model of focus on treating the middle and late stages; reform only treatment and not prevent into prevention and control and treatment at the same equal level.

How to implement this new unification model?

It should be established the hospital of the prevention and control and treatment during the whole process of occurrence and development of cancer .

(2) how to create "the innovative molecular level cancer hospital"? How to implement and create?

Preparations work in two steps:

First of all, rent a house to build the hospital, in order to carry out early work, first try and first start.

Followed by the election area to build a new hospital, about 2-3 years later, it can be fully carried out the work

(1) to build the hospital of the full prevention and treatment with innovative molecular tumor

1	2	11	12
3	4	13	14
5	6	15	16
7	8	17	18
9	10	19	20

1	2	11	12
3	4	13	14
5	6	15	16
7	8	17	18
9	10	19	20

First rent two builds with 6-storey floors to have enough parking spaces
1st floor outpatient   high risk group physical examination
2 floor clinics   rent three years a year to pay a year rent

3rd floor outpatient clinic

4th floor three early

5 floor three early, precancerous lesions

6 floor office, laboratory, school group

Gradually selecting the sites to build a new hospital and there must have enough parking spaces

500-1000 beds, facing the world

Please 1-2 retired Chief Executive Officer, the office director to preside over the preparatory work.

Contents:

- the department of the prevention of cancer and the department of the control cancer, three early outpatient, three early wards, precancerous lesions ... ... and so on

- The establishment of multidisciplinary related groups and laboratories

- Each equipment and the instruction of physical exam and screening (all of the equipments merge with the United States)

- The study project of the prevention of the cancer, three early, precancerous lesions protocol is provided by Professor Xu Ze, Chen Yanchang, Ye Wangyun, Xiang Nan,Li Hangsen, and Xu jie, Chen etc.

- Ask the provincial health committee or a leading cadre of the University of Traditional Chinese Medicine to participate in this comprehensive prevention and control hospital leadership (secretary) and create experience.

Study:

Three early diagnosis: new reagents, new methods, new technology

Three early treatment: new technology, methods, arrangement prescription

Treatment methods of precancerous lesions and observation methods

The Surgery requirements Quality: the prevention of cancer recurrence and metastasis and cultivation need to *start from the surgery, it should attach importance to "Non-tumor technology."*

Non-tumor technology research: it is the requirements of international high level; in China there are more patients and it should be more experience in surgery, excellence, each case are preoperative discussion, postoperative discussion, analysis, regular follow-up.

To create:

1. *Three early study group:*

2. *Precancerous lesion study group:*

3. *Cancer metastasis study group:*

4. *Prevention cancer research group:*

5. *Cancer control Research Group:*

6. *Intravascular "target" organ treatment group:*

Physical examination and screening

The Establishment of Global Demonstration of the Hospital – Prevention and Control and Treatment at the same attention

1. Condense Wisdom

1). Condense wisdom, condense technology, condense high technology and scientific research and integration (mature experience, technology) and condense patents and condense monographs and condense the project topics and condense forward-looking and the exploratory prevention and control and treatment research(Research topics, goals, programs, indicators, outcomes, closely integrated with clinical practice)

2). the cooperation projects and cooperation issues

Put forward a number of topics proposed from the clinical → after experimental study → back to clinical, to solve practical problems→ improve the quality and level of medical care to benefit the patient.

Raised a number of questions, the subject (three early, precancerous lesions, invasion, transfer). To put forward the extisting question is why? Study why? To solve why? How to do? Thus it will be helping to solve the practical problems of clinical care, improve the quality of medical care.

3). to Create:

(1) Medical Research Group - Medical treatment Research group-------medical treatment and research

A. Each case is discussed to study the specific requirements, measures, drugs, techniques and methods to prevent postoperative recurrence, metastasis and anti-complication, and strive for excellence;

B. Adhere to the ward round system, consultation system, preoperative discussion system,

postoperative regular follow-up system

(2) Teaching and Research Group - Teaching Research Group - Teaching and Research - Training graduate students, advanced students, young doctors

(3) The prevention research group-----the prevention and control research group--- the prevention of cancer, cancer control and research should develop the prevention of cancer and cancer control research new areas, new technologies, new industries; should be from the clothing, food, shelter and walking to research the prevention of cancer and to prevent cancer from the big environment and the small environment ; first monitoring, qualitative, quantitative, set the standard, the establishment of multi-project laboratory, the specific methods and measures to prevent cancer.

- Emphasis on improving the quality of medical care, good service attitude, layers of responsibility, adhere to the rounds of the system, preoperative discussion system, postoperative discussion system, discussion and consultation system.

- Responsible system, chief physician responsibility system, physician responsibility system at all levels

- Emphasize wholehearted service for the patient, the urgency of the patient, the pain of the patient, the patient as a loved one, care for patients, care for patients, respect for patients

- Bonus is not linked to medication. Reward and medical quality, service attitude linked, medication, prescription, open check not rebate, not linked with the bonus

- Improve the physician's integrity, respected and reverent

- The doctor should be responsible for the words and deeds, and should be respected by the patient and his family

- Every prescription must have a reasonable theoretical basis for each doctor's advice

- nurses should do care, visit the ward, guide patients with medical care, do not engage in the form, to engage in the actual benefit of patients

- To restore the level of medical care in the 1950s, 1960s and 1970s

- Hospital guidelines should be: to improve the quality of medical care, improve service attitude, to help patients recover

- To restore the physician's rounds at all levels, to fulfill the duties of physicians at all levels.

The chief physician should solve the problem that the deputy chief physician can not solve.

Deputy chief physician to solve the problem that the attending physician can not solve.

The attending physician should solve the problem that the resident can not solve.

Responsible for all levels of responsibility, check,

Layer technology is responsible for, check,

To improve the quality of care

- The department should have the medical routine of the undergraduate course, so that the technology has rules to follow.

- Section director should set the routine, grasp the regular (Section director is the technical director, not only the executive director, should grasp the medical, teaching, research).

- Doctors have a learning system to continuously improve their academic level, technical level and level of diagnosis and treatment

- Have academic reporting system, medical record discussion system, in short, it should pay attention to medical quality, service attitude, academic improvement.

The Establishment of the hospital of the innovative molecular tumors with the prevention and treatment during the whole process

To build the hospital with the prevention and treatment of cancer during the whole process of the development and occurrence ------ the global demonstration hospital with cancer prevention and treatment

---------Selecting the Location of the new hospital

1. The bases:

According to the prevention and treatment of cancer, the strategic thinking of the prevention and treatment of cancer during the whole process of the cancer occurrence and development it is to build a new type of tumor prevention and treatment hospital.

2. The method:

Change the contents of the cancer treatment reform, innovation and development in the third monograph "cancer treatment of new concepts and new methods" into clinical practice; into the implementation in the majority of cancer patients who can benefit. It is the establishment of transformation of medicine and the research and development work group and the establishment of the transformation of medical center and medical is benevolence and the moral legislation is for the first.

3. the planning:

(1) size

① the number of beds prepared

The first stage (1-3 years) 100-300 beds

The second stage (3 years -) 500 beds

The third stage of 1000 beds, facing the world

② the coverage of an area of 15000m2 30000m2 45000m2

(300 beds) (500 beds) (1000 beds)

Have enough parking spaces

(2) the personnel and departments: staffing: medical, nursing, medical technology, prevention, control personnel

1). Outpatient first outpatient second outpatient third clinic

(Specialist characteristics) (specialist focus) (specialist characteristics) (remote outpatient service)

2). Ward (40 beds per ward)

3). The departments

Each department is in charged by a senior professor and a professor of academic academic leaders.

Technology should be domestic first-class

Department of internal medicine, surgery, gynecology, three early, anti-cancer, cancer control, precancerous lesions, radiation diagnosis, ultrasound, electrocardiogram, cavity

mirror chamber room, operating room, pathology room ...

Immunology and Cancer Research Group and Laboratory

Virus and cancer research group and laboratory

Endocrine hormone and cancer research group and laboratory

Fungi and Cancer Research Group and Laboratory

Environmental and Cancer Research Group and Experiment

Three early study group and laboratory

Precancerous lesion research group and laboratory

④ hospital departments set up, set the following multi-disciplinary testing:

A. immunology and cancer discipline

B. molecular biology, cytokines and cancer disciplines

C. virus and cancer discipline

D. endocrine hormones and cancer disciplines

E. fungi and cancer disciplines

F. tumor marker detection, angiogenesis factor detection

G. trace element detection

H. coagulation factor and blood viscosity, blood rheology, thrombosis, anti-tumor bolt test

I. endoscopic examination

J. Ca Cell culture and chemotherapy sensitivity test

K. pathology + immunohistochemistry

L. gene detection

M. carcinogens monitoring

That we build an innovative molecular tumor full anti-hospital is to reform for the overall strategy of cancer treatment and is to change from attention to treatment into prevention and treatment at the same time and the same attention.

After Professor Xu Ze experienced more than 30 years of the cancer basic and clinical research, it was deeply understood:

to achieve the purpose of prevention and control of cancer must start the total attack, that is, the prevention cancer + control cancer + cancer treatment three stages of work imultaneously; three Driving goes hand in hand in order to achieve lower morbidity, improve the cure rate, reduce mortality, prolong survival. If it is only treatment, or heavy treatment and the light defense, it will never be able to overcome cancer. Because it can not reduce the incidence, the more treatment and the more patients.

We have to build "the hospital with the innovative molecular tumor prevention and treatment " is to overcome the cancer to start the overall clinical practice and the prevention of cancer + control cancer + treatment cancer at the same level, to explore a large number of three early diagnosis and treatment, technology, medicine, basic theory of the experiment and new research, to find out new drugs, new technologies, new theories, to find out the new technologies, new drugs, new methods, new methods, new techniques, new theories of the treatment of precancerous lesions. With the current advanced imaging and morphological diagnostic techniques CT, MRI, B sound, etc, once the cancer is diagnosed, it is already in the late, it is difficult for three early diagnosis and treatment. Professor Xu Ze proposed to attack the cancer and launch a total attack which is unprecedented in human work, must create their own experience, must practice in person. This is a new cement road and every step will leave the eternal scientific footprints. Therefore, I suggest that a provincial health and health committee of the Office of cadres as a hospital leadership during the whole tumor prevention and treatment to create experience.

To apply for the preparation of a XuZe plan as shown in the new model of the hospital of the prevention and treatment of cancer during the whole process of the occurrence and development which is unlike now to the invasion of the main model of the hospital. This new type of prevention and treatment of hospital is in close connection with clinical practice and aims for the current problems and shortcomings of the traditional therapy to put forward a series of initiatives and the reform and development and to change in the current global setting up the hospital model with the attention treatment and ignorance of the prevention of the caner.

Anti-cancer out of the way is in the prevention of cancer; the treatment out of the way is in the three early, so it may reduce the incidence of cancer, improve cancer cure rate, prolong survival.

4. Why is it "to build a global demonstration hospital of the prevention and treatment during the whole process of the occurrence and the development of cancer "?

Because in the current in the global and China the cancer hospital or hospital of the Department of oncology are all the hospital treatment model.

1). treatment of objectives : the patients are invasive period, the late patients.

2). diagnostic methods: are CT, MRI, B super ... ... and other advanced technology imaging and morphological footprints; it should have a certain volume, physical, shape in order to show the size of the occupancy; if there is no size of the volume of the entity, the imaging X film can not be shown. Therefore, in the current it is considered that less than 5cm of liver cancer is as "small liver cancer." Therefore, CT, MRI, B sound, although very advanced technology, but once cancer is diagnosed, that is, it is in the late and can not be found early. We must try to study the new technologies of the "three early" diagnosis and treatment.

3). the hospital mode: are the treatment of hospitals with the heavy treatment and light defense, or only treatment .

4). the hospital mode reform: should be changed to the prevention and control and treatment at the same level and attention.

5). the way out of cancer treatment is the "three early": must study the new technologies and the new methods of three early diagnosis and treatment.

Table:

	XZ-C put forward to the hospital model with the prevention and treatment During the whole process of cancer occurrence and development	the current global tumor hospital (treatment Hospital)
hospital mode	prevention+control+ treatment	only the attention of treatment without prevention or ignore defense
The goal or Target	the whole process of occurrence and development	mostly invasive stage or middle and late stage
The objective skills of diagnosis	three early, precancerous lesions foci cancer needs to be studies	CT, MRI,B sound(location and occupany
Treatment	biology treatment and immune Treatment and different induction and surgery treatment and Chinese medication, the combination Of the Chinese and western medications, Laser	surgery , radiotherapy and chemotherapy
The expected Results	can be cured	can not be cured, just ease, in the relief of 4-6 weeks above, then development and metastasis and invasion again
The expected goal	decreasing the cancer incidence rate Increasing the cancer cure rate Can conquer cancer	can not decrease the cancer incidence rate; the more treatment and the more Patients; can not conquer cancer

As mentioned above, the overall strategic reform of cancer treatment should shift the focus or emphasis on treatment to both prevention and treatment.

5. Why is it proposed to build the hospital of the prevention and treatment of cancer during the whole process of the occurrence and development ?

The following is a brief description of the whole process of the the occurrence and development of cancer; it is to clarify the necessity and feasibility of the prevention and treatment during whole process

Cancer occurrence and development experience the susceptible stage and the precancerous lesions stage and the invasive stage. At present, the treatment of cancer in various cancer hospitals or oncology is mainly concentrated in the middle and late stages. The effects of treatment are poor. If the middle and advanced patients can be operated on, they will be treated surgically. If they cannot be operated, they can only be treated with palliative care. Therefore, the way out for cancer treatment is "three early", early detection, early diagnosis, and early treatment. In the early stage, the general treatment effect is good, and the effect of treatment is improved, which will inevitably reduce the cancer mortality rate. Therefore, we must pay attention to the study of early diagnosis methods and treatment methods, but also must pay attention to the treatment of precancerous lesions to reduce the middle and late stage patients in the invasion stage.

Occupying lesion can be seen through CT or MRI, middle or advanced stage

stage of susceptibility	precancerous lesion	early stage	no metastasis	have metastasized	
				local position	amphi position

①   ②   ③   ④   ⑤   ⑥

① Cancer prevention

② Outpatient service of "three kinds of earliness"

③ Surgical operation

④ Place surgical operation first, radiotherapy, chemotherapy and biological TCM second

⑤ Possible to undergo surgical operation

⑥ To give treatment as carcinomatous metastasis

If patients have been treated well in the stage of precancerous lesion or early stage, then the number of patients in middle or advanced stage of invasion and metastasis will fall off. Thus, the cancer incidence rate will also decline. Therefore, we hold that the present tumor hospitals in various places mainly focus on the cancer treatment in middle or advanced stage. Even though the therapeutic result is effective, it can only bring the reduction of cancer mortality rate. But if ignoring the stage of susceptibility, precancerous lesion or early stage, it will be impossible to reduce the cancer incidence rate. Therefore, we must put much emphasis on the whole process of cancer production and growth. After all this is the real global change of strategic importance.

The author has been engaged in oncology surgery for more than 60 years, more and more patients, and the incidence of cancer is also rising, which makes me deeply understand that cancer should not only pay attention to treatment, but also pay attention to prevention, in order to stop at the source. ***The way out for cancer treatment lies in "three early" (early detection, early diagnosis, early treatment), and the way to fight cancer is prevention***.

*As stated above, the center of gravity of the strategic for tumor treatment and prevention moves forward. Its meaning has two aspects: one is **to prevent means such as changing lifestyles and improving environmental pollution**; the other is **to treat precancerous lesions and prevent their progression to the invading or mid-late stages.***

In 1990, the specialist clinic of Surgery Oncology in our hospital opened a "three early" clinic for various endoscopy and biopsy. Many gastric atypical hyperplasia, intestinal metaplasia, atrophic gastritis, breast hyperplasia have been discovered... These "precancerous lesions" are more difficult to treat. How to deal with these precancerous lesions or precancerous conditions to prevent cancer, it is necessary to conduct clinical research and find a good treatment.

Attention should be paid to the research or study of the basic and clinical diagnosis and treatment techniques of precancerous lesions.

The key to cancer treatment is "three early", and how to deal with precancerous lesions is a critical stage in cancer prevention and treatment . The diagnosis of current cancer is mainly diagnosed by the influence of B-ultrasound, CT, MRI and other influences. However, once it is found that it is mostly in the advanced stage, many patients have lost the chance of radical resection. Although comprehensive treatment is done, the effect is still very poor. If the cancer is early or cancer in situ, the surgical treatment is effective and can be cured. Therefore, the treatment of cancer should be "three early", early detection, early diagnosis, early treatment.

Since the pathogenesis of cancer is not well understood, primary prevention of the pathogenesis of cancer is still very difficult.

Recent studies have shown that malignant tumors rarely undergo cancerous changes directly from normal tissues, but before clinical tumors appear, it is often after a fairly long evolutionary phase, which that is the precancer stage. Early identification and control of these precancerous lesions has positive implications for secondary prevention of cancer.

What is precancerous lesion?

The precancerous lesion is a histopathology concept, which refers to a kind of tissues with the dysplasia of cells. Precancerous lesion has the potential to become cancerous. If there is no cure in a long period, precancerous lesion will evolve into cancer. In other words, precancerous lesion just has the possibility of changing into cancer. But not all the precancerous lesions will eventually become cancer. Through proper treatments, precancerous lesions may return to their normal states or have a spontaneous regression.

Canceration is a developing process with several stages. There is a stage of precancerous lesion between normal cells and cancer. It is a slow process from precancerous lesion evolving into cancer, which needs many years or even more than ten years. The length of canceration course is closely related to the strength of carcinogenic factors, individual susceptibility and immunologic function. Therefore, the study of precancerous lesion is of great importance to cancer's prevention and control.

More than one third of cancers can be prevented.

The tumor formation is a long process with several factors and stages. Precancerous lesion is of reversibility, so cancer is preventable.

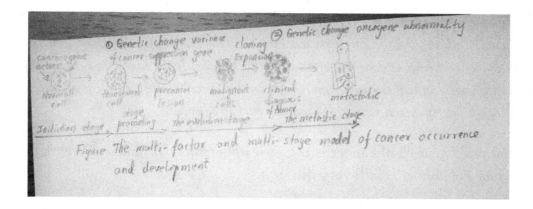

Figure 1 Multi-factor multi-stage model of tumorigenesis

Early primary cancer growth

In the initial stage of primary cancer, *the nourishment of tumor cell growth is provided by infiltration of tissue micro-environment adjacent to the tissue.* The diameter of the tumor at this stage is generally not more than 1-2mm. The number of tumor cells is no more than 10^7, and the pathology is called carcinoma in situ. More clinical reports have been found in cervical carcinoma in situ, esophageal carcinoma in situ, and gastric carcinoma in situ. *In situ carcinoma has a good prognosis after surgery or endoscopic resection.*

The occurrence and development of tumors are experienced in the stage of susceptibility, precancerous lesions and invasive stages. Our current treatment focuses on the invasive stage, the mid-late stage of the tumor. Such a situation is still at an initial level from the perspective of conquering cancer. The key to human terminal control of tumors should not be in the middle and late stages. In the future, it will certainly advance from the advanced tumor to the early stage, precancerous lesions and even the susceptible stage. This is also consistent with **the "Moving forward of Center of gravity for Disease Prevention and Control" strategy** proposed by China's National Medium- and Long-Term Plan for Science and Technology Development (2006-2020).

6. 5-year survival rate of cancer of the status quo is still hovering at a low level in the present in the global

It can be said that today's clinicians in the clinical treatment of cancer options and methods available more and more. But we have to face a reality, a large number of clinical epidemiological analysis shows that the diagnosis and treatment of the ability and means of maturation and development, and the overall effect of tumor improvement seems not fully synchronized. According to the American Cancer Society (The American Cancer Society) data (Figure), nearly a decade, a variety of malignancy diagnosis and treatment level than in the past has been greatly improved, but its 5-year survival rate is still hovering in a Lower level. Such as the 2004 global colon cancer 5-year survival rate of 62%, although the colon cancer diagnostic techniques and surgical treatment has made considerable progress, but only increased to 65%, did not make a breakthrough. Liver cancer etiology, epidemiological studies and a variety of treatment techniques have been greatly improved, but the current 5-year survival rate of only 18%, 10 years ago, only increased by 11 percentage points, how to improve the prognosis of patients is still troubled Hepatobiliary surgeon's problem. The mortality rate of gastric cancer has been high, although the level of surgical technology continues to improve, but the 5-year survival rate of gastric cancer from only 10 years ago, 23% to 29%. In addition, the 5-year survival rate of pancreatic cancer than 10 years ago little change in the 5% up and down; esophageal cancer 5-year survival rate has been maintained at 14%; breast cancer 5-year survival rate from 10 years ago, 87% Down to the current 79%, cervical cancer from 71% to 69%, lung cancer 5-year survival rate from 15% to the current 14%.

The Comparison of 5 - year Survival Rate in Global Malignant Tumor is the following:

At present, most clinicians are more concerned about the specific treatment of cancer and treatment technology research and research, surgery can be bigger and bigger, the treatment program can also be more and more complex, but the lack of cancer etiology of the fundamental means of treatment is a Objective reality.

The diagnosis of cancer is mainly by CT, B ultrasound imaging can only be diagnosed, but once found in the late, many patients have lost the chance of radical resection, although the comprehensive treatment, the effect is still very poor, if Can improve early diagnosis, early cancer or carcinoma in situ, the surgical treatment is effective, can be cured.

Therefore, the treatment of cancer in the early three early, early detection, early diagnosis, early treatment, the prognosis is good.

7. **The stage of applying and preparing the science city (the medicine and the teaching and the research and the development) of conquering cancer**

(1) <u>Why is it I to become the total designer, the President, the Chairman of the General Academic Committee of the "Science Center for Cancer Science"?</u>

<u>*Because all of these total basic assumptions and basic design are put forward by me. Each department (medical school, research institute, hospital, experimental center) is my basic ideas and design and planning and blueprint. I put the purpose, the goal, the task, the method, the step, the scientific research route, the scientific thought, and the preliminary development of the mission of the Science City; I will design the president, the* common dean, executive dean, executive president and vice *president and the task, responsibility and the division of labor clearly and the implementation of their duties; to do their duty, to build. The goal is to achieve results and produce the achievement, unified arrangements and the unified deployment.*</u>

How is this scientific research ship of " the Science City of overcoming Cancer " operated ?how is it to operate these small ship such as Target, course, task, destination? how to plan a boat?

It must be clear the goal to achieve the purpose of conception of cancer and it must be coordinated and be the collaboration; the goals are consistent to overcome cancer and to launch a total attack.

(2) Wuhan anti-cancer research teams of overcoming cancer are the research team which is the combination of the old, middle and young .

① The old age:

more than 65 years old, 70 years of age, 80 or more for the older generation has more than 40 years of rich clinical experience, teaching, research are experienced;

②the middle age: 55-65 years old, more than 30 years of mature clinical experience;

③The Young age: 35-55 years old, with momentum, energy, enthusiasm, is the main, is the focus, you can further development, development, innovation.

(3) New China's medical creation and development is developed by our own.

After the liberation of 1949, the new Chinese medicine is poor and white. *At that time surgery is only to do hernia, hemorrhoids, anal leakage ... ... and other surgery.* In 1951, Peking Union Hospital, Professor Guan Hanping performed subtotal gastrectomy, the surgeon from all of the city visited and observed. After the liberation of 20 years there was no connection with and the United States, Britain, France and other diplomatic relations and it could not study and visit from other countries and no English magazines, books; it all relied on our own self-reliance development and relied on the clinic work after the success in the animal experiments. **The Chinese are smart and hard. In the** *1970s, China achieved many major medical results. In the 60 - 70 years China put a lot of medical satellites and created a medical miracle. Dr. Qiu Caikang in Shanghai Ruijin Hospital saved the 85% area of third-degree* burns; *Shanghai Six Hospital successfully replanted broken arm;the artificial insulin synthesis had the success; Tianjin General Hospital has the half cycle or there was Half-body circulation of Tianjin General Hospital; in Beijing, Xi'an, Nanjing, Henan Anyang the cardiopulmonary bypass had been applied in clinics after the animal experiments or the extracorporeal circulation in Beijing, Xi'an, Nanjing, and Anyang, Henan Province was clinically successful after the animal experiment; In Shanghai Ruijin, Wuhan Tongji liver transplantation was applied for the clinics after the animal experiments ... ... are shocked the world. Chinese people can create miracles in medicine. Go our own way, others have already and we have to learn and have to have; others do not have and we should create our own characteristics or advantages and it should be combined with innovation and international medicine modernization and strive to take our own characteristics of independent innovation path, promote the 21st century and the new development of modern oncology.*

(4) why do I study cancer? I am a clinical surgeon and do the general and chest surgeon work, why do I study cancer? and propose to launch a total attack and to build "the science city of overcoming cancer "?

It is because:

1). in 1985 I conducted the petition on 3000 cases of thoracic and abdominal cancer patients which I operated by my own, the results are found that most patients were the recurrence or metastasis within 2-3 years. *Therefore, we must study the prevention of postoperative recurrence and metastasis methods to improve postoperative long-term efficacy.*

2). I suddenly had acute myocardial infarction in 1991. After the treatment was improved and it was the recovery, it was not appropriate to go to the operating table again. I should not be on the operating table and was to calm down and hid in the small building to concentrate on scientific research.

3). **through experimental studies it was found that thymus atrophy and immune dysfunction are one of the etiology and pathogenesis of cancer and it needed to expand and in-depth study.**

4). through experimental research and clinical validation, after 30 years of more than 12,000 cases of clinical validation observation, **we found the new road of the modernization of Chinese medication in the molecular level of the combination of the Chinese and Western medication with this innovative "Chinese-style anti-cancer" and the new road of Chinese medication immunoregulation to prevent thymic atrophy, promote thymic hyperplasia, protect bone marrow hematopoietic function, improve immune surveillance at the molecular level of combination of Chinese and western medication to conquer cancer so that it persists and continues to study. Therefore, it is proposed to overcome the cancer and to launch a total attack, to build the "Science City" of conquering cancer in an attempt to achieve: reduce the incidence of cancer; improve cancer cure rate; extend the survival of cancer patients; to reach "three early" (early detection, early diagnosis, early Treatment), early can be cured. To achieve the prevention and control and treatment at the same attention . Both Prevention and treatment at the same attention can overcome cancer, reduce the incidence of cancer.**

All basic research must work for clinical and improve patient efficacy so that patients benefit. The evaluation criteria for the efficacy of cancer patients should be:

① *live a long time, extended survival*

② *good quality of life*

③ *no complications - to reduce complications, and even no complications*

Of course, this is only one of the ways to conquer cancer. There may also be vaccines, gene targeting, etc. The roads need to be explored and studied.

Through research on cancer prevention and treatment and putting effort on prevention and control and treatment equally importance or attention, humanity will surely overcome cancer and eventually will overcome cancer.

It should avoid empty talk and pay attention to hard work and start to go. No matter how far away the cancer path is, it always should go. Wanli Long March eventually start going, thousands of miles began with a single step.

1. **Why should we build the prevention and control and treatment demonstration hospital?**

The purpose is:

①**change the hospital mode**

To Change from paying attention to heavy treatment and ignoring the prevention into prevention +control+ treatment at the same attention

② **change the treatment mode**

- *from only treating the middle and late and metastasis and severe ---- poor efficacy, more complications.*

- *change to focus on "three early" precancerous lesions, in situ cancer ----the effect is well and it can be cured*

③ **change the drug cost burden**

- *Late stage, aggressive, metastatic, severe, radiotherapy, chemotherapy, targeted drugs - ---- the cost is high and it uses the expensive medications*

- *Early stage, precancerous lesions, carcinoma in situ, polyps------ it needs the minor surgery + immune regulation or differentiation induction, traditional Chinese medicine, less money, no need to have radiotherapy and chemotherapy, reduce the burden on patients and the state.*

The aims:

①**The way out of cancer treatment is the "three early"**

Anti-cancer out of the way is in the prevention

② the target of the prevention of cancer and anti-cancer and the evaluation criteria are:

To reduce morbidity, reduce mortality, prolong survival, improve quality of life, reduce complications

③What is the results of the treatment of cancer patients?

It usually considered to be:

Patients with long survival time, good quality of life, fewer complications.

2. why should it build the new hospital and the existing top three hospital can not be used?

Because:

①The new hospital mode is the hospital model which the mode has been changed.

The prevention + control+ treatment at the same level and attention and time

To Focus on three early, precancerous lesions, carcinoma in situ, polyps ... ... and so on

<u>The hospitals cannot consider or think of making money as the goal and it should mainly be for the service and public welfare.</u>

The Hospital income is greatly reduced.

② due to focus on three early, precancerous lesions, carcinoma in situ, polyps ... ... and so on, It only needs to have the small surgery, endoscopy ... ... immunotherapy, differentiation induction therapy, Chinese and Western treatment ... ... and so on

Then, the radiotherapy and chemotherapy are not used or greatly reduced.

Because it is early, PET / CT ... ... and so n do not have been used or greatly reduced; CT, MRI greatly will be reduced.

Hospital income is greatly reduced, patients and countries are greatly reduced economic load

③ *For reducing the hospital income, it can be added by improving the diagnosis and treatment fees and the testing technical fees and the surgery costs, etc.*

So it is to try a new demonstration hospital to achieve early diagnosis, early treatment and the combination of prevention and control ad treatment to improve efficacy, prolong survival, improve quality of life, reduce complications, reduce medical costs, reduce patients and Health insurance costs, reduce the severity of patients (because of early detection, early treatment, good effect); due to the good efficacy the doctor-patient relationship is good too.

XZ-C proposed how to conquer cancer I see four:

4. How to conquer cancer? In order to conquer cancer, it must create " the animal experimental center of the experimental medicine cancer"

- in order to conquer cancer, to build "the science city of conquering cancer and launching the total attack" **one**

(1) *Why creates "the Animal Experimental Center of the Experimental Medicine Cancer "?*

① in order to overcome cancer → conquest cancer → capture cancer, we must first understand the basic understanding of cancer clearly :

What are cancer cause, pathogenesis, pathophysiology, immunopathology, and cancer cell biological behavior? What is metastasis mechanism? Why is it implanted? What is the recurrence mechanism?

A series of oncology and tumor-related issues have not yet clear, oncology for scientific research is a virgin land and it needs to be a lot of basic scientific research and clinical basic research. To carry out the basic research of cancer science is the urgent need of the current oncology discipline.

Therefore, we must establish "the animal experimental center of the experimental medicine cancer ".

② *To carry out the basic research of oncology, a good laboratory is the key.* The scientific design, scientific vision, must be finished through laboratory experiments in order to draw conclusions and the results.

We believe that the establishment of the scientific basis (the Science City) for the development of launching the total attack must first vigorously build the laboratory, so that many basic problems have experimental research, open up the basis of tumor research, should encourage the development of new areas of research and produce the talent and the results to help capturing cancer.

③ *to overcome the cancer and to launch a total attack and to build experimental medical cancer animal experimental center, the good equipment laboratory is the key.*

For the study of the new drugs of the prevention of cancer and anti-metastasis it must do the nude mice animal model experimental study. The Experimental surgery is extremely important in the development of medicine and it is a key to open the medical closed area, many diseases prevention and treatment method is applied to the clinical after in many animal experiments it achieved the results of stability and promote the development of medical career.

How can technology have the innovation? How can we overcome cancer? A good laboratory should be built.

*Therefore, for the development of science, scientific and technological innovation and the production of the result and the patent, **the laboratory is a key condition.***

How to carry out basic research on cancer? How to develop new research areas of cancer?

How can the original innovation of cancer research be done? *A good laboratory should be established.*

(2) *How to set up " the animal experimental center of the experimental medicine cancer "?*

The Experimental animal experimental center should not be located in the city center and downtown and it can be located in the suburbs and the University City.

Location: to be in the University City Huangjia Lake

Animal buildings should be enclosed terraces or have enclosed veranda, and the Peripheral or surrounding is isolation.

It should be met to national laboratory requirements management.

The Total Design Blueprint of "the Science City" Of Conquering Cancer and Launching the Total Attack

One of the preparation work of " the Science City"

10. How to overcome cancer? In order to conquer cancer, it must be founded "experimental medicine cancer animal experimental center"

To overcome cancer, it is built the "Science City" by one

How to create "experimental medicine cancer animal experimental center"?

1	7
2	8
3	9
4	10
5	11
6	12

The front view

Closed or lanai   Closed or lanai

The side view

A 6-storey building with closed terraces on each side of the building. It is isolated from the surrounding area and cannot be located in the city center or downtown area. It can be located in the university town on the outskirts of the city.

The recommended points:

Located in the Huangjiahu University of Traditional Chinese Medicine (or nearby)

As a provincial key experimental medical laboratory, according to national laboratory requirements

(emphasizing the importance of cancer animal laboratories, respecting the scientific dedication of experimental animals)

It contains:

(1) Animal model establishment room

(2) Cancer cell culture room

(3) Large animal sterile operating room

(4) Small animal laboratory

(5) Pathology, immunohistochemistry, microscopic examination

(6) Nude mouse laboratory

(7) Postoperative observation room and postoperative ward (cage, cabinet)

(8) Molecular biology laboratory, immunization room, biochemistry room

(9) Laboratory animal breeding room (white mice, rats, rabbits, dogs, monkeys)

(10) Experimental study on precancerous lesions, pathophysiology, pathogenesis, carcinogenesis, invasion, metastasis and prevention and treatment

First laboratory: liver, pancreas, gallbladder, chronic inflammation, virus

(11) Experimental study on precancerous lesions, pathophysiology, pathogenesis, carcinogenesis, invasion, metastasis and prevention and treatment

Second laboratory: stomach, intestinal dysplasia, intestinal metaplasia

(12) Experimental study on precancerous lesions, pathophysiology, pathogenesis, carcinogenesis, invasion, metastasis and prevention and treatment

Third laboratory: women, milk, ER, PR

The experimental medicine:

(1) Experimental animals

Use animal experiments to verify biomedical phenomena, analyze and compare, find rules, and achieve achievements one after another. *It is "experimental medicine."*

(2) Genetic breeding, seed conservation, breeding, feed, disease monitoring, environmental facilities, environmental protection, experimental techniques of experimental animals

Experimental animals are research tools, animal experiments are research techniques

(3) Classification of experimental animals:

1. Inbred animals

2. closed group of animals

3. Hybrid group animals

(4) (4) Experimental animal application:

Animal model of disease:

At present, most biomedical topics rely on experimental animals.

Most of the postgraduate thesis is the result of animal experiments using animal models.

(5) Laboratory animal environment and facilities

The experimental animal environment is related to the health and survival of experimental animals, and it is also related to the value of scientific research and test results.

The experimental animal room is 15-20m² large and small, and the wall and ground structure are suitable.

The temperature and humidity of the animal room should be 18~29°C. Generally, there should be no windows in the experimental animal room, and artificial lighting should be used indoors.

Animal rooms need to be fully oxygenated.

Different animals need different care equipment.

The various feeds required for experimental animals have national standards;

Feeding management and sanitation of experimental animals; feed; cleaning, disinfection and sterilization;

Air conditioning ventilation and lighting; for laboratory animal management requirements, please refer to the Guide to Laboratory Animal Feeding and Management.

(6) Animal experimental surgical operating room facilities and management

It should be an independent building structure, and should not be too close to public places, so as to avoid the noise of experimental animals (such as dogs) affecting the surrounding environment.

The large animal chronic laboratory should meet the standard of the sterilization operating room. The size of the operating room should be 25~45m², and the dressing room, dressing room, instrument room, disinfection room and office should be attached (should be strictly separated from the small animal laboratory). There should be ventilation, sound insulation, oxygen supply, suction device and other equipment. The daily work of the animal operating room is handled by a special person. The head of the animal operating room is responsible for the animal operating room equipment:

a. fixed equipment

It is roughly the same as a clinically sterilized operating room. There should be a large animal universal operating table to suit dogs, monkey, pig, rabbit and other sterilization operations, equipped with a movable shadowless lamp. UV disinfection lamp, instrument table, anesthesia table, Narcotics, medicine cabinets, dressing cabinets, suction devices, infusion sets, oxygen cylinders, oxygen supply equipment, slewing stools, injections, and transportation,For liquid appliances, etc., sterile chest surgery or sterilized abdominal surgery can be performed.

b. Surgical instruments and dressings and preparation rooms.

In addition to the basic surgical instruments that are commonly used, microsurgical instruments, surgical microscopes and microsurgical instruments, as well as cardiac and vascular surgical instruments, and other surgical instruments and special surgical instruments suitable for experimental animals should be prepared. They should be placed in a sorted manner and placed neatly.

Surgical towels and dressings of different sizes should be available to suit the needs of animals of different sizes.

c. Basic equipment for scientific research

Water tank, drying oven, centrifuge, balance, microscope

The experimental study of cancer is mainly the experimental study of cancer cell invasion and metastasis;

Methodology and model establishment of cancer cell invasion research; research on relationship between microenvironment and cancer cell invasion and metastasis; molecular biology research on cancer cell invasion and metastasis; experimental study on anti-invasive and metastatic drugs;

The study related to tumor metastasis, recurrence and clinical practice;

The study related to cancer cell invasion, metastasis and clinical practice;

Experimental Center Scientific Design

Chairman of the academic committee

⎫
⎬ DR. Xu Ze
⎭

Experimental Center Leadership and Academic Committee:

In order to overcome cancer and launch a general attack, "Building a Cancer Animal Experimental Center" is a key to establishing a good laboratory.

Xu Ze (XU ZE) Professor proposed:

- The research on cancer etiology, pathogenesis, recurrence, metastasis mechanism must be carried out experimental laboratory experiments.

- In order to study and carry out effective measures to control invasion, recurrence and metastasis, it is necessary to carry out experimental medical animal experiments.

- In order to find new anti-cancer, anti-metastatic and anti-recurrence new drugs from natural medicines, experimental animal experiments must be carried out to produce animal models of cancer-bearing animals, and experimental screening studies on the anti-tumor rate of Chinese herbal medicines in cancer-bearing animals are carried out.

- How to conduct basic research? How to open up new research areas? How can we produce original innovations?

A good laboratory should be built.

- How can technology be innovated? How can we overcome cancer? It is key to establish a good laboratory.

- The innovative oncology medical school of "The Science City"; the innovative oncology research institute; the innovative tumor prevention and treatment hospitals, **all should be based on their own training of talent, the key is to build a good equipment laboratory. I deeply understand the importance of the laboratory.**

Based on developing and training talents by our own; the key is to build a good laboratory. I deeply understand the importance of the laboratory. I am the first group of college students in the post-liberation college entrance examination. I have not studied or trained outside further or studied abroad, but I have achieved many international achievements. The key is that I have a good laboratory. *I participated in the extracorporeal circulation animal laboratory in the 1960s. In the 1980s, I established the cirrhosis ascites laboratory. In the early 1990s, I established the Institute of Experimental Surgery which was based on conquering cancer as the main direction of cancer.* My animal laboratory has good equipment conditions. There are animal experiments such as mice, rats, Dutch pigs, rabbits, dogs, monkeys, etc. There are better sterile operating rooms for animals, which can be used for major operations in dog chest and abdomen and the animal wards or rooms for observation after the animal post-operation and it can bring various designs, ideas through the experimental operations to achieve results or conclusions.

Therefore, the laboratory is a key condition. If no laboratory passes the experiment, it can only be designed and conceived. It is impossible to become a factual result.

XZ-C proposed how to conquer cancer I see six:

6. How to conquer cancer? In order to conquer cancer, we must create "the innovative molecular tumor pharmaceutical factory" and " the research group and laboratory to analyze the anti-cancer and anti-cancer metastasis active ingredients and the molecular weight and the structural formula and the immunopharmacology at the molecular level"

(1)   Why should we create an innovative molecular tumor preparation pharmaceutical factory and the research group for the analysis of anti-cancer, anti-cancer metastasis active ingredients, Chinese medicine immunopharmacology?

Because it is necessary to research and develop effective drugs for anti-cancer and anti-cancer metastasis, XZ-C believes that it is necessary to have two wheels for cancer, one is the life science, biomedical (modern medicine) **A wheel**. One is the clinical basis, immune regulation, anti-cancer (Chinese herbal medicine) **B wheel**.

Its purpose is to further develop the anti-cancer and anti-cancer metastasis of Chinese herbal medicines, which, and to use the natural medicine as a resource to carry out modern research and make it become precision medicine.

Further study on the molecular level of immunomodulatory anti-cancer Chinese medicine cells.

Further explore the effects of anti-cancer and anti-cancer Chinese herbal medicines on early carcinoma in situ and precancerous lesions.

Its purpose is: in-depth development of Chinese herbal medications of anti-cancer, anti-cancer transfer is indeed effective, removing crude or coarse and keep fine and the natural medicine herbs are as the resources and _conduct the modern research to become precision medicine_.

Further study on the molecular level of immunomodulatory anti-cancer Chinese medicine cells.

Further explore the effects of anti-cancer and anti-cancer Chinese herbal medicines on early carcinoma in situ and precancerous lesions.

(2) _How to create an innovative tumor preparation pharmaceutical factory and analytical group and laboratory of chinese herbal active ingredient?_

Experimental surgery is extremely important in the development of medicine. It is a key to opening the medical exclusion zone. Many disease prevention methods have been studied in many animal experiments, and the stability results have been applied to the clinic to promote the development of the medical cause.

Therefore, the development of science, technological innovation, and laboratories are key conditions. Self-reliance and self-cultivation of innovative talents, the laboratory is the key condition.

11. Prepare a research group and laboratory for the analysis of effective components of anti-cancer and anti-metastatic Chinese medicines.

The aims:

(1) Further research and development of the experimental and clinical study and clinical application of the immune regulation and control of XZ-C anticancer Chinese medicine at the cytokine molecular levels

(2) Further exploration of prevention research and clinical application of prevention cancer and anti-cancer Chinese herbal medicine for early carcinoma in situ and precancerous lesions

Purpose:

In-depth exploration of Chinese herbal medicine anti-cancer, anti-cancer metastasis is indeed an effective drug, to remove crude and to keep fine and remove fake and store real

Using natural medicines and Chinese herbal medicines as resources, modern research is carried out to become a precise medicine.

The methods and the steps:

(1) the animal experiments:

a. in vitro experimental screening

b. in vivo experimental screening

(2) the molecular level experimental study:

The Induction of anticancer lesions differentiation

The anti – cancer and anti - cancer metastasis Chinese herbal medication screening

(3) the gene level experimental study of anti – cancer and anti - cancer metatastosis Chinese herbal medication screening

The topic selection and material selection:

First study from the clinical application of effective Chinese herbal medicine and first separate the active ingredients

The laboratory:

(1) Equipment: Equipment for drug composition analysis

(2) the personnel: the scientific and technological personnel to preside over the analysis of drug ingredients .

(3) The topic selection and the material selection

(4) The expected results

XZ-C proposed that for 30 years we carried out the following series of research work during the process of developing XZ-C immunoregulation anti-cancer Chinese herbal medications:

(1) In the experimental study of exploring the pathogenesis, invasion and recurrence and metastasis mechanism of cancer

From our laboratory experimental results it was found that:

In the cancer-bearing mice the thymus was atrophic atrophy and volume reduction; the cell proliferation was blocked; the mature cells decreased. To the late stage of the tumor, the thymus was extremely atrophic and the texture becomes harder.

From the above experimental study it was found that thymus atrophy and immune dysfunction may be one of the pathogenesis and pathogenesis of the tumor, it must try to prevent thymic atrophy, promote thymocyte proliferation, increased immune function . It should seek immune regulation methods and do the effective drug research from the body's immune function, especially cellular immunity, T lymphocyte function and thymus immune regulation function and explore at the molecular level.

It should further study to find the new ways of cancer treatment and the new methods from the thymus function and tissue structure, immune dysfunction and how to promote immune function so that the immune function can be the reconstructed and how to "protecting the thymus and increasing the immune function".

(2) Experimental study on finding and screening anticancer and anti-metastatic drugs from natural medicines

In our laboratory it was conducted the following the screening tests of the new anti-cancer and anti-metastatic drugs from traditional Chinese medications:

(1) the use of cancer cells in vitro culture method to conduct the screening experimental study of the Chinese herbal medication inhibition rate:

In vitro screening test: the use of cancer cells in vitro culture to observe the direct damage to cancer cells.

The screening test in the tube: In the test tube for culturing cancer cells, the crude crude drug (500 ug/ml) was separately placed to observe whether it inhibited the cancer cells. We conducted 200 in vitro screening tests of Chinese herbal medicines that traditional Chinese medicine believes have anti-cancer effects. And under normal conditions, the normal fibroblast culture was used to test the toxicity of the drug to the cells, and then compare.

(2) *Making animal model of cancer-bearing animal and conducting experimental screening for the screening test of the tumor inhibition rate of chinese herbs in the cancer-bearing animal experiments*

The inhibition test in vivo screening test:

Each batch of experiments consisted of 240 mice, divided into 8 groups, 30 in each group, the 7th group was the blank control group, and the 8th group was treated with 5-FU or CTX. The entire group of mice was inoculated with EAC or S_{180} or H_{22} cancer cells. After inoculation for 24 hours, each rat was orally fed with crude drug powder, and the traditional Chinese medicine was screened for a long time. The survival time, toxicity and side effects were calculated, the survival rate was calculated, and the cancer suppression rate was calculated..

In this way, we conducted a four-year experimental study and conducted an experimental study on the pathogenesis, metastasis, and recurrence mechanism of tumor-bearing mice and an experimental study of how tumors cause host death for three years. More than 1,000 tumor-bearing animal models are used each year. A total of nearly 6000 tumor-bearing animal models were made in 4 years. After the death of each experimental mouse, pathological anatomy of the liver, spleen, lung, thymus, and kidney was performed, and more than 20,000 sections were taken to explore whether it is possible to have a carcinogenic micro-pathogen. Tumor microvessel establishment and microcirculation in 100 tumor-bearing mice were observed by microcirculation microscopy.

Experimental results:

Among the 200 Chinese herbal medicines screened by animal experiments in our laboratory, screening out 48 species did have a certain, even excellent, inhibitory effect on cancer cell proliferation, and the tumor inhibition rate was 75-90%. However, there are also some commonly used traditional Chinese medicines that are generally considered to have anti-cancer effects. After screening in vitro and in vivo, the anti-cancer effect of the animals has no anti-cancer effect, or the effect is very small. This group has been screened by animal experiments and eliminated 152 kinds of no obvious anti-cancer effects.

The 48 traditional Chinese medicines with good cancer suppression rate were selected by this experiment, and then the optimized combination was repeated to repeat the cancer suppression rate experiment in vivo. Finally, the immune regulation and control anticancer Chinese medicine XU ZE China$_{1-10}$ (ZX-C $_{1-10}$).

Z-C$_1$ could inhibit cancer cells, but does not affect normal cells; Z-C$_4$ specially can increase thymus function, can promote proliferation, increased immunity; Z-C$_1$ can protect bone marrow function and to product more blood.

The Clinical validation

On the basis of the success of animal experiments, clinical validation was carried out. That is to establish a tumor specialist clinic and research collaboration group of anti-cancer, anti-metastasis and recurrence with combination of Chinese and Western medicine; keep outpatient medical records, establish a regular follow-up observation system, and observe long-term effects.

From experimental research to clinical validation, new problems are discovered during clinical acceptance, and back to the laboratory for basic research, and the new experimental results are applied to clinical validation.

Thus, experimental-clinical-re-experiment-re-clinical, all experimental studies must be clinically verified, observed in a large number of patients for 3-5 years, and even clinical observations for 8-10 years, according to evidence-based medicine, with long-term follow-up And evaluable information, the evidence clearly has a good long-term effect.

The standard of efficacy is: good quality of life and long survival.

XZ-C immunomodulation anticancer traditional Chinese medicine preparation has been applied to more than 12,000 patients with advanced cancer in 18 years and has achieved remarkable results. XZ-C immunomodulatory Chinese medicine can improve the quality of life of patients with advanced cancer, enhance immunity, increase the body's ability to fight cancer, enhance appetite, and significantly prolong survival.

Now is the fourth stage of our research work. We are carrying out and carrying out research work, step by step, and focus on the research objectives or "targets" in prevention, control and treatment, focusing on the study of "three early" and "precancerous lesions" and further exploring prevention research and clinical application of the anti-cancer and cancer-control Chinese herbal medicine for early carcinoma in situ and precancerous lesions

Exclusive research and development products:

A series products of XZ-C immune regulation and control anti-cancer Chinese medicine (introduction)

(see attached).

12, the preparation for the publication work: the prevention of the cancer and anti-cancer:

Wuhan Anti-Cancer Research Association will publish the following publications and monographs:

1. Popularize prevention cancer scientific research and popular science maps

2. Publishing prevention cancer and anti-Ca popular science books and "People's Medicine" quarterly

3. Publishing magazine publication "Clinical recurrence, metastasis based and clinical" bimonthly

4. Publishing "The Collection of Papers - Cancer Treatment Innovation" monograph

5. Publishing the monograph "tumor-free technology" - how to do cancer radical surgery, anti-recurrence, anti-metastasis

6. Publishing the "three early", "precancerous lesions" publications

7. Publishing the publication, quarterly " Knowledge from clothing and food, housing and walking to prevent cancer"

XZ-C proposed how to conquer cancer I see five:

5. How to conquer cancer? In order to conquer cancer, we must create "the innovative environmental prevention cancer research institute"

---- *One of the science cities to conquer cancer*

(1) Why is it to create an innovative environmental protection institute?

Because: in the current the incidence of cancer is on the rise, which 90% is related to the environment.

The occurrence of cancer is closely related to people's clothing, food, living, walking and living habits.

The current environmental pollution is serious, and the degradation of ecosystems may be related to the increase in cancer incidence.

We have reviewed and reflected 60 years of cancer research work and clinical research and clinical and deeply appreciate the cancer not only to pay attention to treatment, but also to pay attention to prevention; in order to stop at the source, it must do the prevention and treatment at the same time ; the way of out of the anti-cancer is the prevention and the prevention is as the main.

So how to prevent? What is it to prevent? The various environmental carcinogens must be measured, qualitative, targeted, quantified, and sought to remove them.

Therefore, we must establish anti-cancer research institute, should do the prevention research from the clothing, food, shelter, walking and from the big environment and the small environment to the micro, ultra-microscopic anti-cancer research.

How to carry out the prevention cancer research? First of all, it should master and understand the situation of containing carcinogens in the clothing, food, shelter and walking? whether does it contain carcinogens? The qualitative and the quantitative monitoring, and then set the standard, set the bottom line, to discuss and to put forward anti-control measures.

(2) How to set up "the innovative environmental protection cancer research institute"?

The prevention cancer research is a major event and currently the global does not have *prevention cancer research institute*. We will apply that in the Science City of overcoming cancer it is to create "the world's first prevention cancer research institute" to do the macro, micro, ultra-microscopic environmental protection carcinogens monitoring and the analysis to implement the prevention cancer system engineering.

13. How to overcome cancer? In order to overcome cancer, it is necessary to launch a general attack. The general attack is to carry out the three-stage work of cancer prevention, cancer control, and cancer treatment in the whole process of cancer occurrence and development, and carry out simultaneously the prevent, control, and treat. It must pay attention to prevention of cancer. Prevention is the top priority. How to prevent? What to prevent? How to prevent it? This will be discussed in detail below. How to overcome cancer? To overcome cancer, the Innovative Cancer Research Institute must be created or it must create "innovative anti-cancer research institute."

With the improvement of people's living standards, a variety of high-tech products bring us a better life ; at the same time it may also bring a lot of negative effects. A variety of chemical, physical, biological environment, a large number of carcinogens, a variety of carcinogenic substances enter into our human body or a variety of carcinogenic factors affect our body, leading to an increasing incidence of cancer.

Look at the current situation: the incidence of cancer in the status quo is more and more patients, the current incidence of cancer in China is 312 million of the new cases of cancer in the annual incidence and the average daily new cancer patients are 8550 cases and in the country every minute there are 6 Diagnosed as cancer.

Now XZ-C proposed the scientific research programs of conquering cancer and launching a total attack; the prevention cancer and anti-control and treatment at the same level and attention and troika and go hand in hand.

So how to prevent? How to control? What is it to prevent? What is it to control ? How much is it to prevent ? How much is to control? The target or goals of the prevention of cancer or control of cancer must be clear; **a variety of environmental carcinogens must be measured and be qualitative and be quantitative and be positioning.**

Because cancer is thought to be mainly caused by factors such as the environment, diet, hobby and so on; people will attach great importance to the carcinogenic factors in the environment and strive to clear them.

In order to carry out the prevention of cancer and cancer control work, Professor Xu Ze proposed:

(1) it should prevent cancer from the clothing, food, live, walking and from the big environment and the small environment.

(2) it should set up the following anti-cancer research group, please graduate students to carry out and complete the scientific research work.

Professor Xu Ze, as the chief designer, put forward the following research projects and the topics in order to overcome cancer and it must carry out the following research work:

(1) *to understand what needs to be the prevention ? What needs to be controlled? How to prevent? How to control? It must be qualitative and be quantitative and be positioning and be monitoring and be clear and be specific data, we must master the first-hand information in order to do the scientific and accurate anti-cancer work, we must attach importance to the accumulation of raw data, as accurate scientific data and experimental anti-cancer in accordance with.*

(2) *how to achieve this plan and to do his scientific research work? It can be put into the training of graduate students and it can be conducted by the doctoral students, master's degree candidates; it can be both to cultivate the field study of graduate students, but also received anti-cancer, carcinogens qualitative, quantitative analysis* and analysis of components, and further propose anti- method.

The Method:

by the school graduate students to set up the subject and have the purpose and there are tasks arranged arrangements.

(My graduate students is this case, the tutor general subject is like a table banquet, each graduate student is a small sub-title, as frying a dish, Ph.D is frying a large market and the master students is frying a small dish), so give full play to graduate students, but also cultivate the scientific thinking and the scientific and practical ability of graduate students and products out of the paper and products a talent and product a result.

We must pay attention to scientific and technological papers and it is not written by the pens; however it is come from the scientific and technological work. It is necessary to pay attention to the original information, attention to scientific and technological innovation, attention to advanced, innovative and practical. We must pay attention to scientific research and honesty.

How to prevent cancer from the clothing, food, live and walking ? First of all, it should grasp and understand the clothing, food, live, and other crops containing carcinogens; whether it contains carcinogens and the qualitative and the quantitative and the monitoring and then set the standard, set the bottom line, to discuss, put forward the prevention and control measures.

It is proposed to build the following research groups:

(1) The research group : [clothing] clothing, cosmetics and other carcinogens monitoring and prevention and control of cancer:

purpose:

method:

technology:

Equipment conditions:

personnel:

The expected results and achievements: whether there are the carcinogenic substances, qualitative, quantitative, set the bottom line, set the standard micro, ultra-microscopic monitoring;

The analysis and the conclusions: the prevention and control measures are proposed, or it is further to do experiments and to do animal models.

Graduate student (master, Ph.D)

tutor:

(2) [food] food carcinogens monitoring, prevention, control research group → the research Institute

Pickles: pickles, dried salted fish, sausages, mustard, bacon, fermented bean curd, pickles, canned fish ... ... carcinogens content monitoring, qualitative, quantitative micro-research

Fried: ... ... and other carcinogenic content monitoring, the qualitative and the quantitative micro-research

Speculation: ... ... and other carcinogenic content monitoring, qualitative, quantitative micro-research

Smoked: ... ... and other carcinogenic content monitoring, qualitative, quantitative micro-research

Cooking: ... ... and other carcinogenic content monitoring, qualitative, quantitative micro-research

Steaming: ... ... and other carcinogenic content monitoring, qualitative, quantitative micro-research

Smoke stove: ... ... and other carcinogenic content monitoring, qualitative, quantitative micro-research

Leftovers: ... ... and other carcinogenic content monitoring, qualitative, quantitative micro-research

Overnight leftovers: ... ... and other carcinogenic content monitoring, qualitative, quantitative micro-research

Grain: ... ... and other carcinogenic content monitoring, qualitative, quantitative micro-research

Oil: ... ... and other carcinogenic content monitoring, qualitative, quantitative micro-research

Vegetables: ... ... and other carcinogenic content monitoring, qualitative, quantitative micro-research

Meat: ... ... and other carcinogenic content monitoring, qualitative, quantitative micro-research

Fish: ... ... and other carcinogenic content monitoring, qualitative, quantitative micro-research

The supermarkets sell a variety of food (packaged)

(3) [live]: housing, decoration (painting, paint ...) materials, furniture ... ... carcinogens monitoring and the prevention and control research group

Materials, air, microscopic, ultrastructural carcinogens

Whether the excessive (for several large advertising companies ...)

Trace element determination and monitoring

(4) [line]: automobile exhaust, automotive equipment carcinogens monitoring and the prevention and control research group

Cars, trains and other equipment, air

train:

aircraft:

Battery car

(5) Water, pollution (sewage of various factories, air) carcinogens monitoring and the prevention and control research group

(6) Fertilizer, pesticide, soil grain, genetically modified food, whether carcinogens monitoring and the prevention and control research group

(7) whether the computer and the mobile phone have the role of causing cancer or damage monitoring and the prevention and the control research group

(8) the research group of the monitoring of whether air, air conditioning, hood, ray, radiation, nuclear radiation measurement have the carcinogen and the cancer prevention and control

(9) Chinese food, Western food are together with micro-qualitative, quantitative monitoring whether there are the carcinogenic and the qualitative and the quantitative and the standard

- Objective of the study: To determine whether carcinogens and their contents are available, qualitative, quantitative and standard

- Method: Arrange the doctorate, postgraduate program, project

The primary screening and research is to find the problem → ask questions → research problems → solve the problem

Participants: chefs, nutritionists, mentors, graduate students, cafeteria, hotels, restaurants, snack, hot noodles, powder

The researchers come to the scene to study the subject design, experiment, practice to carry out scientific research work

Tutor - graduate - nutrition expert trinity monitoring, research, analysis

- The general arrangement of the subject, the purpose, the request can be a college, responsible for the one hand.

- 100 graduate students, ie 100 papers, preliminary carcinogen composition, quantitative, qualitative monitoring, analysis with funding.

- For the support of the Department of Education, the Office of Science and Technology, the Office of Environmental Protection, the Health and Health Committee

- For college support, guidance, leadership, it will be able to obtain a large number of epidemiology, nutrition disciplines, preventive medicine, public health, environmental science principles of scientific research, to prevent cancer, cancer control first-hand information.

"Three Early" Research

Early diagnosis technology, early diagnosis of reagent research, looking for early diagnosis methods, reagents:

1. *to monitor changes in trace elements:*

Normal: 500 cases

Precancerous lesions: 500 cases

A variety of cancer patients: 500 cases

Various patients: 500 cases

A variety of tumor specimens were cut: 500 cases

Specimens:

blood, urine, saliva, feces, sputum

Inflammatory   neoplasia

Boundary monitoring

Before treatment: After treatment:

2. immune monitoring

Normal: 500 cases

Precancerous lesions: 500 cases

A variety of cancer patients: 500 cases

Various patients: 500 cases

A variety of cancer specimens: 500 cases

A variety of cancer preoperative: 500 cases

Postoperative: 500 cases

Before chemotherapy: 500 cases

After chemotherapy: 500 cases

1   time

2   times

3   times

4   times

Before radiotherapy: 500 cases

After radiotherapy: 500 cases

3. *the endocrine hormone monitoring*

Monitoring of ovarian function and milk Ca: 500 cases

Ovarian function and cervical Ca, ovarian cancer monitoring the search for baseline and bottom line boundaries and monitoring: 500 cases

4. the blood circulation system:

Correlation analysis of hemorheology monitoring and metastasis: 500 cases

Correlation analysis of blood coagulability monitoring and metastasis: 500 cases

Correlation analysis between microcirculation monitoring and micro-cancer or microvascular thrombus embolism: 500 cases

5. the gene system :

1. the analysis of genetic testing is associated with clinical manifestations (symptoms, signs)

2. *the analysis of gene detection combined with pathophysiology, metabolic function, and compensatory function*

3. *Is genetic testing a cause or a consequence?*

Combined analysis and argumentation

6. the study on the combination of tumor markers with clinical analysis and grading

7. CEA ↑ AFP ↑ PSA ↑

It is on behalf of Ca Cells? It can kill cancer? Can it work and be effective? How to handle?

8. the early diagnosis: it is only qualitative, not positioning, how to deal with? What medications are used to deal with?

Printed in the United States
By Bookmasters